Education and Health in Sub-Saharan Africa

A Review of Sector-Wide Approaches

D1716941

World Bank Group
Human Development
Africa Region

Contents

Foreword

Dissatisfaction with traditional project approaches and a recognition of the limitations of the sector adjustment programs led to the development of new lending instruments to improve the impact of development assistance on the sector as a whole. The social sectors have been at the vanguard of these innovations in several countries. Within the Africa Region of the World Bank, the most commonly used such new instrument to provide support for a more comprehensive sector development program has become known as "Sector Investment Program" (SIP).[1] Other agencies have used different names for this approach. For example, under the leadership of the European Union, a group of European bilaterals worked along similar lines and developed a strategy known as "Sector Wide Approach" (SWAP).

In recent years this approach—characterized by a government-led partnership with key external partners, based on a comprehensive sector policy and expenditure framework, and relying on government institutions and common procedures for implementation—has been used by the World Bank for about a dozen operations in the health and education sectors in Sub-Saharan Africa.

This paper is a most welcome review of the experience to date of the Africa Region of the World Bank with this approach. The commitment to Education for All reaffirmed by all partners at the World Education Forum in Dakar, April 2000, and the urgency of an acceleration of education development in Sub-Saharan Africa make the search for more effective ways of working together for education development an inescapable imperative.

This is especially important as the Bank[2] and several bilateral agencies have explicitly indicated their intention to use this approach to channel their support for education development. While the SWAP is not without problems and is not suitable in all countries, some adaptation of the SWAP is likely to become the most important instrument used by external agencies to support accelerated education development in the Africa region. This paper summarizes the lessons we in the Africa Region have learned so far, identifies the strengths and weaknesses of this approach, and provides advice and guidance to operation staff in the Bank, partner agencies, and governments who will be involved in sector-wide approaches in the years to come.

This paper was prepared by Richard Johanson under the supervision of Adriaan Verspoor, Education Lead Specialist in the Africa Region of the World Bank, with the assistance of Angel Mattimore.[3] Con-

---

[1] Peter Harrold wrote the definitive explanation of sector investment programs in his work "The Broad Sector Approach to Investment Lending," World Bank (1995).

[2] See The World Bank (2000) "A Chance to Learn: Knowledge and Finance for Education in Sub-Saharan Africa," forthcoming.

[3] The findings, interpretations and conclusions expressed in this paper are entirely those of the author and should not be attributed in any manner to the World Bank, its affiliated organizations or to the members of the Board of Executive Directors or the countries they represent. The World Bank does not guarantee the accuracy of the data included in this publication and accepts no responsibility for any consequence in their use.

tributions to the paper and case studies were given by Arvil Van Adams, Anwar Bach-Baouab, Rosemary Bellew, David Berk, Nicholas Burnett, Francois Decaillet, Linda Dove, Birger Fredriksen, Donald Hamilton, Bruce Jones, Julie McLaughlin, Paud Murphy, Eliezer Orbach, O.K. Pannenborg, Robert Prouty, Jee Peng Tan, and Steve Weissman (all of the World Bank). We would like to thank the Norwegian Government for providing financial support for the preparation of this study through the Norwegian Education Trust Fund. For more information about this book, send an e-mail message to afrhdseries@worldbank.org.

Birger Fredriksen
Sector Director, Human Development
Africa Region, The World Bank

Summary of Main Points

Project assistance in Africa has been criticized as fragmented, donor-driven and lacking impact on basic development problems. In view of the wide-spread limitations of projects, in the early 1990s a new lending approach was developed in Africa—the "Sectoral Investment Program". The main rationale for this kind of sector-wide approach was to address weaknesses of the project approach and achieve greater impact with development assistance. The main characteristics of SIPs are as follows:

Partnership
- ❖ Local stakeholders in charge—program directed by government
- ❖ All key donors sign on to the program
- ❖ Government coordinates donors
- ❖ Broad consultation with stakeholders

Comprehensive sector policy framework
- ❖ Sector-wide scope, covering all relevant areas, policies, programs, and projects.
- ❖ Based on an (a) overall policy for the sector (principles and objectives); (b) strategy of measures to achieve policy objectives over the medium term (about 5 years); and translated into (c) a program of specific interventions in the near term (2-3 years).

Expenditure framework
- ❖ Overall expenditure program, including definition of feasible intersectoral allocations
- ❖ Intrasectoral spending plan, derived from program priorities

Management systems and capacity building
- ❖ Common implementation structures and procedures (harmonization of donor procedure—including reporting, joint annual reviews of performance, procurement, disbursements to the extent possible)
- ❖ Use and strengthening of government institutions, procedures and staff (rather than external technical assistance)

Sector-wide programs emphasize a process by which overall policies are translated into strategies and programs, then into expenditure plans that make sense in a long-term national context. This is followed by annual reviews of actual performance against the plans and adjustments as appropriate. The emphasis is on process rather than products. Sector-wide programs can be served by different lending instruments, including specific investment loans (SILs), sector investment and maintenance loans (SIMs), adjustable program loans (APLs), and Technical Assistance Loans (TALs).

Innovations in sector-wide approaches include:
- ❖ Policy development as a dynamic process, not a one-off exercise, to be updated and renewed as circumstances become clearer or change.
- ❖ Linkages with the macroeconomic framework. Resource allocation is derived from an overall expenditure framework.
- ❖ Clear linkages established among analysis, policy development, strategic plans, pro-

grams, budgets, and implementation through annual reviews.

❖ The emphasis on harmonization of donor procedures.

❖ The emphasis on use of government structures and procedures for such functions as procurement, financial management, and accounting.

FINDINGS FROM THE REVIEW ABOUT SECTOR-WIDE APPROACHES

In the second half of 1999 a review was conducted in the Bank's Africa Region of sector-wide approaches in the social sector. The intended audience of the review was Bank operational staff in the education sector of the Africa region. The review sought to answer the question: how should a sector program be done? Based on staff interviews, a literature review, and development of eight case studies the findings suggest that a sector program should:

❖ Be developed only in countries that meet the preconditions. (Chapter 1)

❖ Establish an effective collaborative process—which requires a) developing donor-government partnerships, b) following the national leadership, and c) forging donor coordination. (Chapter 2)

❖ Establish a proper policy framework – which requires (a) adopting an appropriate scope, (b) basing it on strong analytical work, (c) consulting with stakeholders about priorities, and (d) continuing the policy development process during implementation. (Chapter 3)

❖ Prepare an overall expenditure framework that (a) defines appropriate intersectoral allocations, a feasible resource envelope, and (b) ensures appropriate allocations within the sector; (Chapter 4) and

❖ Establish management arrangements that (a) analyze and build institutional capacity, (b) concentrate on effective monitoring and

evaluation, and (c) set up appropriate financial mechanisms. (Chapter 5)

It is still too early to tell whether sector-wide approaches in the social sector are making an impact, but some useful findings can be identified.

Sector programs are complex. They involve broad scope, new procedures, donor coordination, and channeling of external assistance through government budgets and the implementation of major reforms. Each of these adds a layer of complexity. Complexity comes at a price—in terms of time and resources required for sector approaches. Different kinds of staff are required, particularly those adept in policy analysis and negotiation.

STRENGTHS

Sector approaches have achieved several successes. Comprehensive plans and strategies were developed in all cases reviewed and in some countries capacities were built for decentralized planning. Stronger links were forged between policies, the allocation of funds and performance. Stakeholder consultations were strengthened and frameworks were established for donor coordination. Some common procedures were adopted by donors, particularly for joint missions, monitoring, and progress reporting. These steps helped reduce the administrative burden on governments of external assistance. Some programs have begun to move to budget support by pooling external resources and channeling them through the government budget. Resources allocated for the sectors have also increased under sector programs in both absolute and relative terms.

WEAKNESSES

Weaknesses identified at the design stage include the lack of rigorous sector analysis in some cases; the lack of systematic analysis of implementation capacity in most cases (such institutional analysis can be an antidote to overly ambitious programs), and inadequate design of monitoring indicators. During implementation, problems and changes are the rule rather than the exception. This underscores the need for doing better risk analysis and contingency planning. Other specific problems have been weak data collection, and disappointment with the outcomes of joint semiannual reviews.

RECOMMENDATIONS FOR BEST PRACTICE

The review concludes with recommendations for best practice and a list of prerequisites for commitment of funding to sector programs. They are reproduced below from the main text:

A. Meet the Preconditions for Starting
   ❖ Ensure that the prerequisites are met for entering into the development of a sector-wide approach. Do not undertake a sector-wide approach unless the client has (a) a modicum of stability, (b) strong commitment to an integrated, collaborative process, and (c) at least a minimum level of institutional capacity. In addition, ensure that the donor agency allocates adequate resources and the right profile of staff for developing a sector program.

B. Establish a Collaborative Process
   ❖ Do not rush the process of policy development. Sector approaches are a long haul, not a quick fix. Time must be allowed for reaching agreements on policy issues and interventions, appropriate procedures, legislation and clear delineation of responsibilities to ensure sustainability (Jespersen: 12)
   ❖ Recognize that success ultimately depends on the level of trust among partners. Trust, in turn, is based on openness, transparency, negotiation, and compromise. Appropriate mechanisms must be in place by which all

parties can raise and address problems and their concerns.
   ❖ Follow government's lead, but ensure that ownership and participation is increased progressively from a narrow group of reformers and includes participation of central ministries and legislatures.
   ❖ Spell out the rights and responsibilities of all parties on paper at the start in a Statement of Intent, and later in a Memorandum of Understanding (or Credit Agreement) and Code of Practice.
   ❖ Harmonize procedures that are feasible immediately, such as reporting, joint reviews, and monitoring systems. Also start with immediate steps to strengthen and improve government systems. Get central agencies to work on generic systems for all sectors, such as finance and procurement, rather than repeating the work sector by sector.
   ❖ Define the role of a donor lead agency in advance to avoid misunderstandings. Provide sufficient administrative funds to pay for the high costs of coordination.
   ❖ Establish a joint technical assistance fund for project preparation to start pooling of resources on a small scale.

C. Establish a Comprehensive Policy Framework
   ❖ Distinguish between sector-wide scope for analytical and for investment purposes. That is, start with a comprehensive policy framework covering the sector as a whole even if subsequent investment programs have to be limited to particular subsectors.
   ❖ Help build stronger analytical underpinnings for sector-wide programs by improving the quality and rigor of sector analysis during initial program design.

❖ Recognize that policy analysis is an important ongoing function during program execution and focus attention on (i) building local capacity for continuing policy analysis during implementation, and on (ii) building better information systems for data collection.

❖ Continue the good work shown on stakeholder consultation. Widen the consultations beyond the bureaucracy to include front-line service workers and beneficiaries. Use a clearly defined resource envelope to ensure realism and facilitate hard choices among competing priorities.

❖ Have explicit policy agreement on basic principles and priorities before loan approval, an explicit list of policies on which consensus has not yet been reached, and a process for reaching consensus through further study and dialogue. Use an adaptable program loan (APL) with "triggers" set for achieving consensus on difficult areas of policy.

D. Develop Financial Parameters

❖ If it is not possible to invest in the sector as a whole, nonetheless monitor expenditures sector-wide to ensure reasonable intrasectoral allocations.

❖ Conduct public expenditure reviews before commitment of funds to establish an overall resource envelope for the sector. Do not defer this to the implementation phase.

❖ Use budget ceilings to force better selection of priorities, as when regions prepare sectoral programs.

❖ Devote attention to the establishment of sound government criteria and procedures for appraisal and selection of specific investment projects.

❖ Meticulously plan the flow of funds from the center to regions and districts to avoid the typical delays in disbursements.

❖ Where other donor funding is uncertain establish a core program of donor assistance with Bank financing, and add to the core as additional financing materializes.

❖ Use computer models for expenditure projections during preparation and use the same models during implementation for monitoring performance.

❖ Spell out the role of the lender of last resort. In particular, agree in advance on what specifically is excluded from the expenditure plan.

❖ Accept "patchwork" arrangements— where donors earmark funds for particular components—only as a step toward the optimal strategy, which is the pooling and channeling of donor funds through normal government budgets.

E. Build Management Systems and Capacity

❖ Use existing techniques for institutional analysis more systematically and rigorously to identify and address weaknesses and constraints before embarking on a sector program. Go beyond organizational analysis to consider staff incentives, identify who stands to gain and lose from program implementation, and plan in detail the flow of funds to beneficiaries. Since institutional analysis is costly, budget the requirements separately and fully in project preparation. Consider using an APL to overcome structural constraints for later phases.

❖ Focus early and sharply on the development of monitoring and evaluation systems. Limit the number of indicators to priorities and ensure that they tell clearly whether the program is on track annually.

❖ Design joint review procedures in advance and ensure that workable mechanisms are in place to identify, address, and resolve problems. Build government capacity to manage joint reviews.

❖ Involve financial and procurement specialists early in the design phase to help in developing appropriate systems.

❖ Link disbursements to achievements to provide incentives for good performance.

❖ Engage in better risk analysis and contingency planning for various types of occurrences. Think through systematically what would happen if critical changes happened in (a) the macro-environment, e.g., if macroeconomic shocks reduce sectoral allocations below planned targets; (b) disagreements arose on the policy framework; and (c) key staff changed. Devise a set of courses of action for each contingency. For example, assuming that key personnel inevitably will change, (i) broaden the participation of stakeholders, (ii) provide continuous training and briefings for new personnel involved, (iii) involve higher levels in the approval process, e.g., cabinets, and (iv) root the programs in legislation. Devise and install remedies at the design stage in case things do not work out and the program deviates markedly from the plan.

❖ After tapping other sources for financing studies and reviews, be prepared to finance substantially larger-than-normal budget coefficients for supervision of sector programs, recognizing that ongoing analytical work is costly to review and the scope of sector-wide programs encompasses the equivalent of multiple projects.

The net effect of these recommendations is to expand the list of actions that must be completed before loan or credit approval, making the preparation process for a development program even more demanding than a traditional project. In summary, the following steps should be considered as *essential prerequisites for commitment of funding* (i.e., in place by time of Board presentation) for sector-wide operations:

(1) *Policy framework developed*, based on rigorous sector analysis, including specific three-year work program (Ethiopia education).

(2) Wide *consultations with stakeholders* and donors have been held, and agreement reached on priorities.

(3) *Public expenditure review* or social sector expenditure review completed; overall *financial parameters defined* in terms of targeted intersectoral allocations and a *budget envelope* for the sector, and agreement on *budget priorities* for the first two years (Ethiopia health).

(4) *Institutional capacity analysis* completed and agreement reached on early implementation of a program to fill identified gaps (The Gambia education).

(5) *Monitoring indicators identified* that show clearly whether program implementation is on track; *data collection system designed* and in place on processes, system delivery and impact (Ghana health).

(6) The modus operandi designed for *joint reviews and problem resolution*, i.e., mechanisms for common reporting, joint annual reviews of progress, budget planning, discussion of differences.

(7) The role of *donor of last resort clearly spelled out* (and specifically what is excluded from the agreed expenditure program), and a staged *plan to achieve pooling* of resources among donors.

(8) Risk analysis prepared as a basis for *detailed contingency planning* for changes in (a) the macro-environment; (b) the policy framework; and (c) key staff. As part of the contingency planning, remedies should have been defined for noncompliance

with, or substantial deviations from, agreements.

(9) Provision of the *correct profile of staff and adequate resources* (including outside financing and internal budgets) for program supervision.

The following are other *desirable but not essential conditions* for commitment of funds:

(1) Donor agreements reached on pooling of resources.

(2) Financial incentives included for good performance.

(3) Harmonization of procedures for financial management and procurement (likely to be a medium-to-long-term goal).

CHAPTER 1

INTRODUCTION

SITUATION

Primary enrollments in Sub-Saharan Africa have not kept pace with population growth. The gross enrollment ratio in primary education declined from 78 percent in 1980 to 72 percent in 1990 before recovering to 74 percent in 1995. (Verspoor:17) In the 1980s spending on education per inhabitant decreased by a catastrophic 65 percent in Sub-Saharan Africa (UNICEF: 13). At the current rate, nine countries are projected to have fewer than half the eligible children in primary school by 2015, including Ethiopia, Mozambique, Angola, and Sierra Leone (Oxfam: 57). Three-fourths of the world's out-of-school children by then will be in Sub-Saharan Africa.

PROJECT ASSISTANCE

The impact of development assistance generally has been disappointing. A study in 1994 by the Bank's Operations Evaluation Department found that 60 percent of all Bank projects in Africa in 1992 were not meeting their objectives. More broadly, project assistance has come under increasing criticism by both donors and recipients. Project assistance in Africa has been criticized as (a) fragmented, (b) donor-driven, and (c) having weak impact on solving basic problems at the sectoral level. These three topics are discussed below.

(a) Project assistance has tended to be fragmented. Many countries host a multiplicity of donor-financed projects. In the agriculture sector in Zambia at one point there were over 145 separate projects. The situation was similar for the education sector in Mozambique, as explained in Box 1.1. Project assistance is often characterized by the lack of use, and the lack of development, of government institutions and procedures. Each donor agency tends to follow separate procedures for the implementation of their projects. For the most part each project requires the establishment of a separate organization (project implementation units) to execute the project in view of weak capacity within normal government structures. This disperses government capacity over many small units (Harrold: 3-4). The net result may well be a duplication of efforts (Cassels: 8-9). The concentration of attention and funds on specific projects also means myopia: lack of an overall view of the sector as a whole, and lack of attention to overall policies, institutional and economic environments, and constraints under which projects must operate (Cassels: 7).

(b) External assistance tends to be donor-driven. Donor agencies typically have their own sets of priorities and kinds of components they would most like to finance. Donors often foist these agendas upon the recipients. The assistance may be based on inconsistent visions (Jones: 24) and conflicts may arise between the different approaches. Donor dominance with parochial agendas can re-

BOX 1.1
Multiple Donors for Education in Mozambique

Prior external assistance to the Ministry of Education was provided under more than 150 different projects and subprojects, by more than 16 countries, 6 UN agencies, 3 major multilateral financing institutions (IDA, African Development Bank, and European Union), and a large number of local and international NGOs operating throughout the country. The Government was simply unable to monitor this large number of projects. In addition, there were serious inequities under these projects in resource allocation to schools, districts and provinces, and more important, resources were often not geared toward urgent priorities. In addition, the numerous project implementation units and independent, parallel activities such as audits, supervision, etc. drew heavily on the limited Government capacity, thereby reducing the Government's resources to undertake their administrative function. This was compounded by the use of different procedures and financial management systems by donors in parallel operations.

Source: Mozambique education case study.

sult in the distortion of spending priorities by subsectors and between types of financing (e.g., development vs. recurrent spending). Donor projects can also tend to be overly designed and overly complicated in a misguided search for perfection or to meet the developed-country standards of the contributing agency. This can result in inconsistent and inequitable standards for an enclave within the education system. Projects with high standards (referred to sometimes as "gold-plated") can be costly or impossible to sustain in poorer countries. Donor-driven projects also tend to be inflexible when faced with changed circumstances (Cassels: 8-9).

(c) Despite successes in individual projects, the consequences of project-based assistance have been weak performance and impact at the sectoral level. (Jones: 4) Harrold (3-4) refers to "islands of success in a sea of failure." The failures can be attributed in large part to the characteristics of projects. Myopic, enclave-type approaches ignore the lack of coherent sector policies, systems and

budgets. The fragmentation strains government systems and personnel. (Peters and Chao: 180-81). It allows shifts in government spending to non-priority items through "fungability." (Jones: 4).

PROGRAM ASSISTANCE

Program assistance (i.e., support for overall programs rather than more specific projects, often on a fast-disbursing basis) has proved to be helpful in particular circumstances, such as emergencies. However, the impact has been limited on sector-wide problems. There are two main types of program assistance, support for structural adjustment and sectoral adjustment, as follows:

(a) Structural adjustment operations (or "SALs") have been able to achieve large, rapid injections of money into countries in crisis. Funds are disbursed in tranches in response to compliance with policy conditions. Structural adjustment has been particularly effective in improving balance of payments (Peters and Chao: 180; Cassels: 9). However, structural adjustment operations typically do not get deeply enough into sectoral issues (Harrold 3-4). They lack long-term horizons, and do not usually control how funds are spent within sectors. Consequently, they have been less effective in promoting long term sectoral objectives (Peters and Chao: 180-1).

(b) Sectoral adjustment operations[1] (or "Secals") were a phenomenon largely in response to the crisis of the 1980s. Most Secals took place between 1985 and 1995. Secals have had mixed success. The sectoral adjustment operation in Guinea showed that under certain conditions (specifically, strong consensus and government support) the lending instrument could lead to increased expenditures for education. More recently, the Uganda Education Sector Operation (February 1998) has had good success in supporting the government's drive for universal primary education. However, as indicated by other operations[2] increased financing for the sector does not necessarily translate into better output or products. As Cassels (p. 9) stated for the health sector, "There is little to be gained by merely guaranteeing funds for an inadequate and inefficient health system." The weakness of sector adjustment operations is that they focused almost exclusively on increased finance for the sector, and did not get deeply enough into programs for improving sector outputs and performance.

THE DEVELOPMENT OF SECTOR-WIDE APPROACHES[3]

The Roots of Sector Investment Programs (SIPs)

Dissatisfaction with project and program approaches led to the development of innovations to improve the impact of development assistance on the sector as a whole. The major development for the Africa Region was the introduction of the "Sector Investment Program", or "SIP," in 1994. Peter Harrold has written the definitive explanation of SIPs in his work: "The Broad Sector Approach to Investment Lending" (1995); Andrew Cassels has prepared the best set of guidelines on sector programs: "A Guide to Sector-Wide Approaches for Health Development: Concepts, Issues and Working Arrangements" (1997).

SIPs draw on earlier experiences outside the Africa region. First, they include elements from more traditional "sector loans", or sector investment and maintenance loans. These (a) focused on policy changes, (b) financed a time slice of an investment program, and (c) delegated selection and implementation of subprojects to intermediary organizations within agreed criteria and procedures.[4] The Tanzania Integrated Roads Project in particular followed this pattern. Second, SIPs are patterned after innovative operations in the South Asia region in which donors agreed to support a common program to raise expenditure in particular social sectors. The Pakistan Social Action Program (SAP) is an example of coverage of multiple subsectors, health, education, and water supply. The Bangladesh Health Program targets one sector.

---

[1] Sector adjustment operations are similar to structural adjustment inasmuch as they disburse funds in tranches on the basis of compliance with policy conditions. They differ in scope, focusing on one sector rather the economy as a whole.

[2] Examples include the Ghana education sector adjustment credits, "EdSAC".

[3] Terminology: The working group under the Special Program for Africa has adopted the term "sector program" to describe the genre. This replaces the terms Sector-wide Approach ("SWAP"), Sector Investment Program ("SIP"), Sector Development Programs (SDPs), etc. However, this review uses the terms "sector-wide approach", "sector-wide program" and "sector program" interchangeably.

[4] See Thomas (1994) and Johanson (1985).

SIP Characteristics

The "Sector Investment Program" is not a lending instrument per se. It is a comprehensive approach that can be supported by an array of lending instruments, including specific investment loans (SILs), sector investment and maintenance loans (SIMs), and—more recently—adaptable program loans (APLs.) Table 1.1 shows the types of lending instruments used for the eight SIP cases presented later in part II of this review.

The main rationale of for the SIP is to address the weaknesses of projects and achieve greater overall impact with development assistance. The presupposition is that sectoral goals can be achieved better through a sector-wide approach and nationally defined policies, strategies, and budgets rather than a series of specific projects (Cassels: 12).

Different reviewers have compiled lists that identify different characteristics of SIPs (Harrold: 6; Jones: 8-9; Cassels: 11; EU: 3) In synthesis, there seem to be four main features, as follows:

(1) Partnership
   ❖ Local stakeholders in charge–program directed by government
   ❖ All key donors sign on to the program
   ❖ Coordination of donors by government
   ❖ Broad consultation with stakeholders
(2) Comprehensive sector policy framework
   ❖ Sector-wide scope, covering all relevant areas, policies, programs, and projects.
   ❖ Based on an (a) overall policy for the sector (principles and objectives);

(b) strategy of measures to achieve policy objectives over the medium term (about 5 years); and translated into (c) a program of specific interventions in the near term (2-3 years).
(3) Expenditure Framework
   ❖ Overall expenditure program, including definition of feasible intersectoral allocations and the resource envelope
   ❖ Intrasectoral spending plan, derived from program priorities
(4) Management systems and capacity building
   ❖ Common implementation structures and procedures (harmonization of donor procedures)
   ❖ Use and strengthening of government institutions, procedures, and staff (rather than setting up parallel systems and using external technical assistance)

Essentially, sector-wide approaches such as the SIP emphasize process rather than products. They emphasize processes by which policies are translated into strategies and programs, then into expenditure plans that make sense in a national and long-term context, followed by joint reviews of actual performance against the plans, and adjustments as appropriate. Sector-wide approaches get away from the idea of finite stages, such as a design stage followed by a full-fledged investment program (Cassels: 13). The emphasis shifts from meeting *ex ante* standards to tracking improvements over time (Grindle: 5). Sector programs do not define everything in advance as does a project. Therefore the processes—especially

TABLE 1.1

Case Studies by Type of Lending Instrument

Lending Instrument	SIP Examples
Specific Investment Loan (SIL)	Ethiopia Health; Ghana Health; Senegal Health
Sector Investment & Maintenance Loan (SIM)	Zambia Health; Ethiopia Education
Adjustable Program Loan (APL)	Gambia Education; Zambia Education
Technical Assistance Loan (TAL)	Mozambique Education

the instruments for dialogue and agreement—become of overriding importance. As noted in several of the cases, e.g., Ghana, a sector-wide approach does not have the security of a traditional project where content and quantities are defined in advance. Instead, the security must be implicit in the procedures by which decisions are made during implementation.

INNOVATIONS IN SIPs

There is much new in this approach, both in absolute terms and relative emphasis, as follows:

(a) Clear linkages are established among analysis, policy development, strategic plans, programs, budgets, and implementation through annual reviews (Peters and Chao).

(b) Policy development is not a one-off exercise, but a dynamic process to be updated and renewed as circumstances become clearer or change (Cassels: 35).

(c) Explicit connections are forged with the macroeconomic framework. Resource allocation is derived from an overall expenditure framework.

(d) Donor procedures are harmonized.

(e) Rather than bypassing normal government institutions and processes, SIPs aim at using and improving government structures and procedures for such functions as procurement, financial management, and accounting.

Sector-wide approaches have attracted a wide range of interest. Many donors, particularly European bilateral assistance agencies, see the approach potentially as a major improvement over project lending. The Nordic countries, the Netherlands, and the United Kingdom have been instrumental in studying and promoting the approach. In addition the EU-convened conferences on sector-wide approaches and the U.N. Special Program for Africa adopted sector-wide approaches as a main theme

for improving assistance to the poorest countries in the health sector.

Within the Bank a growing number of SIPs have been approved and the pipeline is populated with intentions to do more. Most SIPs have been used in low-income, aid-dependent countries with multiple active donors (Zambia, Mozambique, and Ethiopia mainly). The social sectors account for about half of all SIPs. Within this context the health sector has led in the development of sector-wide approaches (for example, the Zambia health sector program was regarded as a SIP retroactively). Increasingly, SIPs are being used in the education sector, including Ethiopia, The Gambia, Mozambique, and Zambia. Problems have also been experienced in the development and implementation of sector-wide approaches. These include client policy changes inconsistent with the agreed framework (Zambia health, possibly Ethiopia); bilateral financing inconsistent with the agreed framework (Ghana health); difficulties of procedures for procurement and financial management (nearly all countries.)

PURPOSE OF THE REVIEW

It is still too early to learn much from implementation experience, but in view of the number of sector-wide operations already in existence, the number of new ones planned, and their potential it is nonetheless important to seek some tentative conclusions. Of necessity, these lessons will have more to do with design than implementation. Therefore, a review was conducted in the second half of 1999 of experience to date, mainly in the Bank's social sector of health and education. The intended audience of the review is Bank operational staff in the education sector of the Africa region. The review sought to answer the question: how should a sector program be done? What does doing a sector program "right" look like?

The review used three sources of information. First, the myriad studies on sector programs were reviewed. (See bibliography for works consulted.) Second, interviews were conducted with task team

TABLE 1.2

Case Studies in the Review

Health Sector	Education Sector
Ethiopia Health	Ethiopia Education
Zambia Health	Zambia Education
Ghana Health	Gambia Education
Senegal Health	Mozambique Education

These appear in Part II of the review.

leaders and other knowledgeable persons within the Bank about sector-wide programs. (See list in Annex 1 of World Bank staff interviewed.) Third, eight case studies of health and education projects were prepared, as shown in Table 1.2.

FINDINGS

Based on the findings of the review, a sector program should :

❖ Meet the preconditions before starting program development. (Chapter 1)
❖ Establish an effective collaborative process—which requires (a) developing donor-government partnerships, (b) following the national leadership, and (c) forging donor coordination. (Chapter 2)
❖ Establish a proper policy framework— which requires (a) adopting an appropriate scope, (b) basing it on strong analytical work, (c) consulting with stakeholders about priorities, and (d) continuing the policy development process during implementation. (Chapter 3)
❖ Prepare an overall expenditure framework that (a) defines appropriate intersectoral allocations, a feasible resource envelope, and (b) ensures appropriate allocations within the sector; (Chapter 4) and
❖ Establish management arrangements that (a) analyze and build institutional capacity, (b) concentrate on effective monitoring and evaluation, and (c) set up appropriate financial mechanisms. (Chapter 5)

These points are discussed in sequence below, followed by conclusions and recommendations (Chapter 6).

CHAPTER 2

MEETING THE PRECONDITIONS
TO START THE PROCESS

A key question is: where are sector-wide approaches appropriate? Where can they be used? In what types of countries is this approach most suitable? The early development of SIPs stressed the importance of meeting various, extensive pre-conditions. However, concern has now shifted from "preconditions" to a more flexible approach based on a common vision by stakeholders with no particular blueprint for implementation arrangements (Grindle: 1).

It is important to distinguish between preconditions to *start the development of* a sector program, and preconditions for *approval of financing.*[1] A basic precondition for starting a sector-wide approach is dissatisfaction with current conditions, e.g., the ineffectiveness of project lending, the system is in crisis. Beyond this, preconditions for starting to develop a sector program boil down to stability, commitment, and minimum institutional capacity:

- Stability. This means two things: (1) Macro-economic stability. There is consensus that it makes little sense to develop sector programs in the absence of a suitable macro-economic framework, i.e., manageable budget deficits, low inflation rates (Harrold: 20-21). The reason is that sector programs need adequate, stable financing. These requirements cannot be met under conditions of high inflation or excess deficit spending (Okidegbe: 3); and (2) Political stability. It

is unlikely that a long term program can be developed or sustained in a context of rapidly changing regimes. The importance of ownership and capacity limits the application of sector-wide approaches to stable environments (Jespersen: 3). As stated in the Ghana health case, " A sector-wide approach cannot be done in a 'stop and go' context."

- Commitment. Sector-wide approaches are defined by intent rather than pre-existing achievements. (Cassels: 14) The main requirements are intent to take an integrated approach and commitment to a collaborative process (EU: 7). This was done quite clearly in two of the case studies: Zambia Health and Ethiopia Education.

- Institutional Capacity. The country must have *at least the minimum level* of institutional capacity to handle the development and implementation of the program. This is a relative rather than normative standard. Of course, institutional capacity can and should be developed further during the program, but some minimum basic capacity must exist to enable the start of a successful process. As Harrold stated (22), "There is a tension between requiring good capacity to exist as a basis for a SIP, and using the SIP process to develop this capacity."

---

[1] Preconditions for financing a sector program are presented in Chapter 7, Conclusions and Recommendations.

These three criteria suggest that sector-wide approaches are not appropriate in all countries. They would not be appropriate where political and economic instability have not been achieved (e.g., in conflict situations or perhaps in recent post-conflict countries). They should be avoided where there is insufficient interest by the client in taking leadership of the process (Peters and Chao: 180).

For example, the failure to develop a health sector program in Cote d'Ivoire can be attributed to inadequate government commitment. Some observers would go so far as to suggest that sector programs are only appropriate for countries with solid implementation capacity and that only a few countries are therefore ripe for sector-wide approaches.

CHAPTER 3

ESTABLISHING A COLLABORATIVE PROCESS

Establishing an effective collaborative process requires (a) developing donor-government partnerships, (b) following the national leadership, and (c) forging donor coordination. These topics are presented sequentially below.

DEVELOPING DONOR-GOVERNMENT PARTNERSHIPS

A sector-wide approach requires a fundamental change in the way organizations behave and relate to each other (Peters and Chao: 180). It involves both adoption of a partnership between government and donor agencies and close coordination among the donors. Some observers feel that success in sector programs ultimately has more to do with the character of the partnership than the technical soundness of policies (Peters and Chao: 186).

Trust, mechanisms for negotiations, and flexibility by participants are key characteristics of successful partnerships. First, trust plays an important role. Sector approaches delegate a significant degree of authority to the recipient country. The donor trusts that the recipient will act in accordance with agreed criteria and procedures. Openness is extremely important for building and maintaining trust. This clearly prevails in the Ghana health program. In contrast, trust has been lost in the Zambia health program (See case studies). Appropriate mechanisms must be established for discussion of issues and negotiation of solutions. Give-and-take is an important requirement for success in partnerships. Decisions must be carefully scrutinized by all parties. Once agreement is reached, all parties assume collective responsibility for subsequent achievements and failures (Cassels: 13).

Partnerships can be threatened by lack of communications (EU: 13), lack of transparency and clarity (Peters and Chao: 186; Jespersen: 4). One of the most significant barriers to effective partnership is frequent conflicts and changes of personnel (Peters and Chao 190). It seems ironic, but almost axiomatic, that once a sector program has been approved—usually involving major institutional and policy reforms—the key personnel on the government or donor side change. These changes disrupt program continuity and explain slow initial implementation in several cases (e.g., The Gambia education).

Experiences of those involved in the process state clearly that it takes time to build partnerships. Stability on both donor and government sides is important. Contingency plans should be made for staffing changes, such as by broadening the consultation process to ensure a wide range of people are familiar with the content and processes of the sector programs.

Finally, it is essential to design appropriate forums for dealing with problems (Peters and Chao: 186). As noted in the Ghana case, it is highly important to have a system in place through which the views of all parties can be aired and disagreements resolved. In the end it is not so important that disputes and differences occur as long as a process of mutual consultation is in place and methods have been agreed in advance on how to resolve disputes and solve problems.

USING NATIONAL LEADERSHIP TO BUILD OWNERSHIP AND SUPPORT

Reviews by the Operations Evaluations Department (OED) consistently point to the importance of national ownership and commitment in ensuring the success of development assistance (for example, the 1994 OED review of 1992 performance.) One overriding aim of a sector-wide approach is to ensure country ownership of the product (Harrold: 23). National leadership is one essential means to ensure ownership of programs. (The other is broad consultation, discussed later.)

Under a sector-wide approach national leadership (or sponsorship) is indispensable for the development of a program. The case of Zambia education exemplifies this point (see case study). The process of developing a sector program foundered in the mid-1990s until a strong, new minister of education took leadership of the process. Then developments fell into place.

Some of the findings on leadership include the following points: First, there is a tendency for leadership and ownership to be vested in a small group of individuals (Jespersen: 4) In most cases SIPs are driven by a few key proponents in the sectoral office. The lack of broad support can lead to implementation problems or delays (Jones: 10, 22; Utz: 7.) Another potential problem is lack of involvement by central ministries, such as the finance ministry, in the process of formulating the sector program (Jones: 22.) Furthermore, the level at which ownership resides is important. For example, the whole cabinet approved the Bangladesh health program, ensuring broad support. If the cabinet or parliament does not approve the program, the program may be in for tough sledding during implementation. It is also important for participants to have clearly in mind in advance which groups stand to gain or lose from the sector-wide approach, as this affects the degree of political support and their viability (Cassels: 29-30). A sector-wide program tends to strengthen the power of senior policymakers and reformers. It decreases the power of individual project managers and other donor-funded fiefdoms and may, therefore, lead to resistance from those quarters. More broadly, sector-wide programs subject the government to greater external scrutiny. Issues that previously were the sole prerogative of government get placed on the agenda for open discussion. Authoritarian regimes could resist this tendency.

Finally, the exigencies of national leadership and partnership need to be reconciled. It is not donors, acting in concert, imposing their agenda on government. Nor is it government authoritatively dictating terms to donors. The government is the final arbiter, but all parties have rights and responsibilities (Cassels: 13). One recommendation from best practice is that these rights and mutual responsibilities should be spelled out at the start in a "Statement of Intent" adopted by all parties, and later in a "Code of Practice" (as was done in the Ghana health case).

FORGING DONOR COORDINATION: WORKING TOGETHER UNDER GOVERNMENT LEADERSHIP

Until donors learn to work together external assistance cannot be fully effective. Sector-wide approaches ensure that all participants share one common set of aims and tell a consistent story. The essence of a sector-wide approach is that donors give up the right to select which projects to finance in exchange for a voice in the process of developing the broad sectoral strategy. Donor-specific project planning is replaced by negotiating how resources are spent within the sector. A joint review of sector performance replaces the evaluation of discrete projects (Cassels: 12).

Donor coordination means two things: (a) agreement on a common program; and (b) adoption of common procedures. Each is explained separately below.

Common Program

The adoption of a common, shared program ensures that all participants aim at the same objectives and means, even though they may be financing different parts. This benefits all parties by eliminating duplication and avoiding parallel, often contradictory, donor-driven designs (Harrold: 12).

Signing on to a common program has several important implications for the partners. First, it means exclusion, that is, agreement by donors not to finance expenditures outside the agreed framework and for governments not to accept financing of things that fall outside the framework (Jones: 24). The case studies show examples in which exclusion was not observed by government (e.g., urban hospitals in the Ghana health program). It is understandably difficult for a government to turn down grant financing of a project with a willing donor, but concentration of resources on agreed priorities demands it. The exclusive nature of the agreed program has to be recognized explicitly in advance. Second, adoption of a common program may mean retrofitting or phasing out existing projects that are inconsistent with the program (Utz: 8). Third, it requires that all participants be completely open and do not try to conceal activities (Grindle: 7-8). It also means that donors are able to assure the government on the timing and levels of their support. This has proved to be problematic. Finally, success is no longer the achievements of particular projects or particular donors; it is shared by all participants for the sector as a whole.

Common Procedures (or "Harmonization")

Adoption of common procedures has been one of the main aims, and one of the main obstacles, for sector programs (Grindle: 5). Adoption of common procedures requires donors to compromise on their own internal procedures, which has proved difficult (see the Ghana case.) The objective of common procedures is to reduce the administrative burden placed on government by different procedures and from donor to donor. The benefits of harmonization are better-quality information, more timely information, reduced duplication and waste, and release of time of government staff (Jespersen: 8).

Harmonization has proved easiest to achieve in four areas: (a) reporting formats and timing, (b) common performance indicators, (c) joint missions, and (d) procedures and norms for technical assistance.

Harmonization is most difficult to achieve in (a) procurement and (b) financial management. Under procurement, the "rules of origin" may prevent multilateral agencies from cooperating. For example, the membership of the World Bank and the African Development Bank are not congruent and, consequently, common eligibility rules cannot be followed. In practice, several donors allege that harmonization in practice means following the standards of the most restrictive donor, or bilateral agencies agreeing to accept the standard procedures of multilateral organizations such as the World Bank (Grindle: 7-8). Financial management is particularly sensitive for all donors. It involves the greatest risk of waste or misapplication of funds. It is also where the gulf between requirements and actual practice is the widest: between requirements for strong accountability by donors and the practices of relatively weak national systems of financial management.

Harmonization of procedures such as procurement and financial management are not usually sector-specific. Much of the work on harmonization could therefore be done beyond the sectoral level (Jespersen: 8; Jones: 34, 41). The parallel development of sector programs in education and health in Ethiopia, with education approximately six months ahead of health, allowed the health sector to use generic procedures developed for education. (See case studies.) The advice from best practice is that central authorities should be in charge of developing common procedures applicable to a range of sectors.

Several factors work against harmonization (Peters and Chao: 184). These include "attribution", or the need for donors to be associated with specific inputs or components (i.e., "showing the flag.") Narrow commercial interests, such as tied procurement, also run counter to the adoption of common procedures (Harrold: 12). Resentment and jealousy often exist between donors, for example at the real or imagined dominance by certain donors including the Bank. Donors must also work through the loss of direct control over the use of their funds. Other obstacles are the inability of some donors to finance recurrent costs, and their inability or unwillingness to change their practices to accommodate new joint methods. Finally, there is the natural tendency of donors not to get overly involved in components that they do not finance. There is a natural reluctance for donors not to criticize others. In the Zambia education case, questionable assistance by one European bilateral donor was tolerated until the sector approach brought all assistance under external scrutiny and discussion. Its low cost-effectiveness was immediately questioned.

Instruments for Coordination

(a) Lead agency. One way to achieve coordination is for donors or the client to appoint a "lead donor." The role of the lead donor is to ensure an open flow of communication among the donors, call meetings, establish agendas, and follow through on actions. Jones (25) has emphasized the importance of a lead donor for reasons of efficiency. Having a lead agency is not essential, but it can make communications more efficient, particularly for the government. For example, a lead agency can reduce the transaction costs for the government in dealing with multiple donors. If a lead agency is selected, best practice suggests that the role, responsibility, and authority of the lead donor be defined in advance and agreed on by all cooperating partners (see, for example, the Mozambique education and Ethiopia education cases.) The World Bank does not need to play the role of the lead donor (see the Senegal health case.) In fact, in only three in the eight cases reviewed was the Bank was the lead donor. One of the issues in having a lead donor is that few donors appear able or willing to delegate fully to the lead agency (Jespersen: 9).

It is clear from experience that the lead donor is likely to incur a heavy administrative burden. The transaction costs are high. In both the Ethiopia and Zambia education cases, the task managers stressed that one cannot do too much donor coordination. Harrold (12) suggested that there should be burden sharing in view of the high administrative costs of coordination. This was in fact done in the case of the Bangladesh health program and the Pakistan SAP by allocating administrative funds explicitly for the purpose of donor coordination units. These helped prevent an endless flow of paper.

(b) Mechanisms for coordination. Several instruments are cited in the literature and the case studies as means of facilitating cooperation among donors.

(1) "Statement of Intent"—these serve to set the parameters for the sector approach and donor coordination at an early stage. Statements of intent ensure that all parties (government and donors) have the same vision of what is intended and expectations. It reduces confusion during program development (Cassels: 52).

(2) "Collaborative Work Programs—set out the tasks, sequence and responsibilities.

(3) Joint missions—in which multiple donors participate to accomplish common terms of reference at the same time in the country.

(4) Joint aide memoires—in which joint missions adopt a common set of findings, conclusions, and recommendations.

(5) "Memorandum of Understanding"—these are usually agreed upon at the stage of commitment of funds (and are often patterned after the Bank's Development Credit Agreements.) They cover topics including: (a) financing—purposes for use of funds; eligible expenditures, commitments on levels, (b) disbursements—how donor funds will be channeled, common accounts, pooling, responsibility for management, readiness criteria government eligibility for pooled funds, (c) procurement, (d) negotiations, consultation, and information exchange—mechanisms for negotiation when circumstances change, timing of government reports, joint

reviews, and exchange of information (Cassels: 53-55).

(6) "Code of Practice"(Cassels: 55) covering such topics as open sharing of information, use of joint missions, and use of external technical assistance only as an exception. This instrument has been controversial[2] and has been slow to gain acceptance. A "Code of Practice" is not a guide for day-to-day decisions, but it can provide a useful reference in cases of disagreements. It is one element in the mechanism for resolving disagreements.

---

[2] For example, one early version of a code of practice stipulated that local and external technical assistance should be paid the same.

CHAPTER 4

DEVELOPING A POLICY FRAMEWORK

A policy framework is the set of policies used by the government to direct the sector. The process of developing a sector program should start, as Cassells (37) wrote, by setting out the big picture about desirable characteristics and essential features of sector delivery. The aim is to establish a minimum set of clear principles for development of the sector upon which strategy can be based (Harrold: 8).

Three levels of definition are involved in a good policy framework:

- ❖ *Policy* (overall goals and principles)
- ❖ *Strategy* (objectives and means to achieve the overall goals, usually with a time frame of 5-10 years); and
- ❖ *Program*, a set of specific measures to implement the strategy over the short to medium term.

Development of the policy framework typically follows the progression of moving from the general to the specific, i.e., from principles to strategy to program. The case studies clearly depict this sequence, including Ethiopia education that moved from overall goals to a program action plan (PAP). The Ghana health project also progressed from overall principles into a focused program of work (POW). The Senegal health project included a similar progression, as shown in Box 4.1.

One of the main purposes of a policy framework is to provide a basis for establishing priorities for public expenditures within an overall resource envelope. It provides a reference for the extent to which expenditure programs support the implementation of sector policies (Jones: 20; Harrold: 8; Cassels: 36).

Some of the findings of the review suggest that reaching agreement on the sector policy framework is more likely the extent to which the sector is in crisis, the narrower the range of institutions involved, the fewer the donors, and the less contentious the topics included (e.g., basic health or education.) Agreement on the policy framework inevitably takes time and involves compromises on the part of donors and governments alike. Donors should resist pressures to accelerate the process (Jones: 29, 38).

Four main requirements exist for the establishment of a workable policy framework: (a) definition of appropriate program scope; (b) strong analytical underpinnings; (c) consultation with stakeholders; and (d) a flexible, ongoing process. Each is explained in turn below.

REQUIREMENT 1:
DEFINITION OF APPROPRIATE PROGRAM SCOPE

An early key decision in the planning process is to define the scope of the sector for which the program will be prepared. According to Harrold (6) the sector should be comprehensive to avoid fragmentation of planning and implementation that could reduce efficiency and output. By definition, a sector-wide approach should avoid being insular and dealing only with certain enclaves. It should deal with relationships between subsectors and components of the system, and between recurrent and capital expenditures.

BOX 4.1
Program Development in Senegal Health

(1) The National Task Force first agreed on an action plan for the design of the program. (2) The second step was to undertake a series of studies to assess human resources, health financing, hospital reform, primary health care, and cost recovery. Donor funds were readily available to finance these studies. (3) Third, based on the findings the Task Force developed a "Long Term Strategic Vision for Health Development." (4) Fourth, the Task Force then developed a 10-year National Health Plan, which identified critical priorities and implementation mechanisms with technical support from multilateral and bilateral donors and involving extensive consultations with stakeholders. Government ownership of the design process was strong with Ministry of Health (MOH) being the driving force behind the process. (5) The long-term plan led then to the preparation of a "Five-Year Action Plan" that spelled out immediate priorities and investment requirements. (6) The Ministers of Health and Finance convened a roundtable of donors at which the Plan was reviewed by donors and pledges were made for the financing of the Plan. This resulted in a well-conceived financing plan, including both national and external sources. (7) Program appraisal came right after the roundtable. Key program documents (strategic framework /long-term plan /and medium-term expenditure program) were reviewed and commented on by donors at regular intervals in the program design process and officially endorsed at the roundtable. There were few disagreements of a substantive nature. Differences centered mainly on administrative and financial procedures.

Source: Senegal health case study.

One suggested criterion for the definition of sectoral scope (Harrold: 7) is whether the program covers the most significant expenditures, i.e., includes all important sector-related expenditures. However, completeness (i.e., avoidance of fragmentation) has to be balanced with institutional feasibility. Jones (17-18) suggests that the key question in deciding scope is whether the program is linked to a clear budget entity for financial management. In effect, the sector program becomes a ministerial program. What should be avoided is a program that is based on cross-cutting themes, such as women in development or even nutrition (Cassels: 20). Such thematic programs cut across too many administrative boundaries to be readily implementable.

Harrold (8) wrote that an education sector program that failed to include tertiary education could not be regarded as a sector program, nor could a program that only included tertiary education. However, comprehensive scope confronts two problems

in education: inadequate consensus on policies at higher levels and weak capacity to manage all subsectors. There is not much agreement internationally on appropriate policies for upper levels of the education system, particularly higher education and vocational education and training. Inclusion of these subsectors in the scope of sector programs could well delay progress on other priority areas such as basic education. Another problem concerns limited government capacity, which would suggest limiting the scope of programs. A recent review of SIPs in Africa for all sectors found them to be characterized by lack of sector-wide coverage. Zambia education (BESSIP) is an example of a decision to limit coverage, as shown in Box 4.2.

Focusing on one subsector, e.g., primary, has appeal from the viewpoint of designing a manageable program. However, dealing with one subsector alone also has potential disadvantages, including: (1) neglect of intersectoral resource allocations leading to critical imbalances between major spending categories; and (2) concentration of donor funds and subsequent unsustainable financing for one level (Cassels: 19; Peters and Chao: 185-86).

In this context it is helpful to distinguish between a sector-wide scope for analytical purposes and for investment purposes. For analytical purposes, a broad definition of the sector is important as a context for defining a coherent framework for sector policy objectives. This provides an overall umbrella for more specific investment work. For investment purposes, it may be appropriate to define the sector more narrowly. The APL instrument provides Bank staff with the opportunity to support a series of subsector programs over time within an agreed sector policy and financial framework. The Mozambique education case exemplifies a sector-wide analysis followed by investment concentrating on basic education.

The conclusion is that a broad sector policy framework should be developed for the sector as a whole in all cases to ensure that the parts of the system are properly placed and dimensioned, even though the investment program may necessarily deal

with only one subsector. Similarly, if it is not possible to adopt a sector-wide investment program, one must nevertheless monitor the overall expenditure framework and track funds at the sector level to ensure reasonable intrasectoral allocations (Peters and Chao: 186; Cassels: 19). The reason is to avoid "fungability", i.e., to prevent external funds from freeing up resources for allocation to activities of low overall priority. This was not done in the Zambia education case.

REQUIREMENT 2:
STRONG ANALYTICAL UNDERPINNINGS

A sector-wide program needs to be built on the basis of thorough sector analysis, including identification of priority issues, causes and consideration of alternative solutions and strategies. Quality sector work is a good predictor of success of a sector program. Harrold referred to Mozambique health as a sector program emerging from good sector work. Another example, drawn from the case on Ethiopia education, is shown in Box 4.3.

BOX 4.2
Deciding on Scope in the Zambia Education Program

The development of this program went through several stages of reduction in scope to achieve a final definition of the "sector," or in this case, "sub-sector." Initially an attempt was made at developing a comprehensive Education Sector Investment Program (ESIP), coordinated by an ESIP Secretariat. Higher education was excluded from the beginning on the basis that it was an area of lower priority for new investment, and the intractable nature of the problems at that level. Even without higher education ESIP still included four ministries, (i) the Ministry of Education; (ii) Science Technology and Vocational Training; (iii)Youth, Sport and Child Development, and (iv) Community Development and Social Services. In September 1997 the Government agreed to divide its program into two financing packages, one for basic education (BESSIP) and another for training (TSSIP)—to be started in about three years. Several agencies are nevertheless involved in BESSIP, including the Ministry of Education, The Public Welfare Assistance Scheme, and a Micro-Projects Unit attached to the Ministry of Finance and Economic Development that will administer community-implemented school construction activities.

Source: Zambia education case study.

BOX 4.3
Strong Analytical Underpinnings for the Ethiopia Education Program

The high level of sector analysis was one of the reasons for Bank acceptance of the sector-wide approach in the education sector in Ethiopia. Annual public expenditure reviews and a social sector expenditure review were available. In particular, the 1997 public expenditure review by the Bank established a medium-term expenditure framework. The bulk of the analysis that preceded the preparation of the Program was produced and facilitated by a Policy and Human Resources Development (PHRD) grant and executed by the Government. The studies developed by the project generated primary data through household, institutional, and community surveys and combined this with secondary data from previous studies. The majority of the work was carried out by local staff and consultants. Nine separate studies were produced, including access to and supply of educational facilities; demand and supply of educational manpower; private and social returns to education; demographic analysis and population projections; household demand for schooling; the role of NGOs and the private sector in service delivery; costs and financing of education; community consultation and participation; and cost effectiveness of key educational inputs. In addition, the Bank's Task Team Leader spent considerable time with other donors to assemble analyses done by other agencies. In particular, USAID, the EU (on higher education) and Swedish International Development Cooperation Agency (SIDA) (cost effectiveness of different types of school construction) had significant studies and analyses that had not yet been widely disseminated.

Source: Ethiopia education case study.

This review found that much of the sector analysis in the cases was ad hoc and not subject to high standards of quality assurance. Most sector work consisted of specific studies financed from project preparation funds and identified after the broad policy framework was already defined. These studies typically were not subject to rigorous quality reviews. The Task Team Leader or local preparation leader were the ultimate clients for the studies. Staff noted that locally conducted sector studies for Zambia education were of poor quality. In some cases the government did not even await the results of the studies to inform its policies before forging ahead (Ethiopia health). In another extreme case, all needed sector analysis and expenditure reviews were done after the commitment of funds for the program (Zambia health).

This raises a question: since a sector-wide approach is a process, why does the timing of the analytical work matter? Analysis is a continuing process.

Surely sector studies can be done later as a basis for refinement and amendment of policies. This is correct, but when the analysis occurs is still important. The analysis first has to provide a basis for initial broad choices of priorities and strategies on which funds will be expended. If mistakes are made in strategy, misallocation of funds inevitably result. The lack of broad, rigorous analysis of issues and alternatives at the start of program development is a cause for serious concern about the validity of programs. Continued analysis is also needed during program implementation to inform the continuous development of policy.

REQUIREMENT 3:
CONSULTATION WITH STAKEHOLDERS

A broad national involvement is necessary to develop a sector policy framework, including beneficiary feedback[1] as an input to policy development. The sensitivity of policies adopted and their likely widespread impact on the population demands consultation. A key to success is the vehicle used to generate national consensus on policies. Involvement of community organizations is important for reaching a diversity of delivery approaches suited to the needs of people. This is especially important given the long-term (10- to 15-year time horizon) involved in the policy framework (Jespersen: 5).

The findings of the review suggest some guidelines for consultation. First, the purposes of the consultation need to be differentiated. Consultation to provide input into design for the policy framework is quite different from the public relations that might be necessary to sell a program to the public that has already been adopted (Jones: 23; Cassels: 31). It is the former that is discussed here. Second, it is important for the government to organize the consultation, not donors. African ministers of education have noted a tendency of aid agencies to try to drive the process of strategy development, including consultation (EU: 9). Third, effective consultation is difficult and often does not get planned properly. There is a tendency to limit consultations to the bureaucracy, as was done in the case of the Ethiopia education and health, rather than front-line workers and beneficiaries. The involvement of civil organizations often appears ad hoc and unstrategic (Jespersen: 5). Fourth, the timing of consultations is important. It should not be done too early, for example, not before the definition of a concept paper and a structure for determining priorities (Harrold: 10), or some tentative priorities and a resource envelope (Jones: 23). Harrold (8) singles out the Zambia agricultural SIP as particularly exemplary for the wide consultations held. All eight cases prepared for this review involved consultation with at least some stakeholders, but in most cases it was fairly limited.

REQUIREMENT 4:
A FLEXIBLE, ONGOING PROCESS
OF POLICY DEVELOPMENT

What distinguishes sector-wide approaches from earlier interventions is that policy development is not a one-off exercise, but a continuing process (Peters and Chao: 192). Typically, policy development is seen as a discrete stage that produces a product—a policy document—once and for all (or at least for the next five years.) The sector-wide approach stresses that policy development is a continuous process. Allowances must be made for refining, changing and adapting policies based on in-depth studies, experimentation and even international experience (Cassels: 35-36; EU: 9). The initial policy statement is important, but it cannot be the last word. If too much attention is paid to its development, time is wasted and reality gets replaced by documentation (EU: 9). Moreover, comprehensive analysis has limits. Everything cannot be analyzed at once. It is easy to miss some topics. For example, the Ghana health program is based on extensive analysis, but did not cover private health care and only now is beginning to fill this gap.

Requirements for a strong process of ongoing policy development include: (a) efforts to build local analytical capacity continuously; (b) experimentation among strategic alternatives and evaluation of the results; and (c) strong performance indicators and monitoring of policy effectiveness so as to inform revisions and adjustments. These requirements, in turn, often place a priority on building better data and information systems.

Often some policy issues cannot be resolved before loan approval. More study and negotiation may be needed. The question is whether sufficient agreement exists between all parties on basic principles and policies to enable a successful start for the sector program. No absolute guideline can be given on what

---

[1] Caveat: it is not possible to include all private sector and NGO institutions (Harrold: 25).

is "sufficient agreement." This has to be decided by authorities in each case. What helps is to be explicit about the policy differences; to agree on the steps, process, and timetable by which the policy issues will be examined in depth; and to outline several courses of action if agreement is not reached. The Adaptable Program Loan affords an excellent instrument to deal with unresolved policy issues. As seen in several cases (Zambia education and Mozambique education), the first phase of the APL focuses on priority activities for which there is consensus. Unresolved issues (e.g., vocational training and higher education) are deferred until later phases. Criteria, or "triggers", are spelled out for moving from one phase to the next. If consensus cannot be reached, subsequent phases would be deferred or substantially reformulated.

CHAPTER 5

DESIGNING APPROPRIATE FINANCIAL PARAMETERS

Sector approaches are distinguished from their predecessors by placing the sector within an appropriate financial context. This involves two aspects: first, ensuring appropriate intersectoral allocations and defining a resource envelope, and second, ensuring correct allocations within the sector. In general, sector approaches seek increased overall funding for the sector and allocation of the increased financing to priority activities. These two aspects are dealt with separately below.

SETTING THE SECTOR WITHIN THE MACROECONOMIC FRAMEWORK

As stated in the introduction, the project approach to external assistance suffers from the weakness of insufficient sustainability. The recurrent cost implications of all projects are not aggregated and fit into an overall framework of what is affordable. Moreover, the project approach suffers from lack of impact on increasing the overall level of allocations to the sector. The sector approach addresses these problems by defining a feasible overall resource envelope and targeting increases in the share of public resources going into the sector. Financial flows to any one sector cannot be isolated from allocations to other sectors.

Determining the total resources available (i.e., the "resource envelope") over the medium to long term is usually done through an overall public expenditure review (PER) (Okidegbe: 7-8). The Ethiopia health and education programs were both based on rigorous analysis of overall public allocations for

the social sector. As stated in the previous section, the preparation of sectoral spending programs involve, or should be preceded by, dialogue with government and civil society about intersectoral priorities for public spending.

Appropriate allocations to the sector can be achieved either by specifying a minimum relative share of public resources for the sector, or by estimating absolute amounts required. Earmarking proportions of government budget for the sector is almost invariably the approach used. All eight cases prepared for this review included targets for resource allocation, particularly Ethiopia education; Mozambique education; Senegal health; and Zambia education. More broadly, sector programs have targeted and increased the funds available for the respective sectors in almost all countries (Peters and Chao: 183). Donors withheld aid in the Pakistan Social Action Program when government did not meet spending targets for social sectors (Peters and Chao: 190).

One common problem in constructing an appropriate resource envelope is how to ensure that all sources of revenue and spending are covered, including private sector contributions. A total picture is frequently missing, owing to weaknesses in financial information and the channeling of donor resources outside normal government accounts (Jespersen: 9; Peters and Chao: 186-87). Another problem has been a weak link between the sectoral approach and other reforms, such as civil service reforms (Jespersen: 6). There is a risk in poor countries in targeting a relative share of the budget. This may result in funds falling short of requirements. In addition, earmarking shares of revenue for one sector can lead to distortions. Sector approaches could distort overall patterns of public expenditure and threaten stability by increasing the level of funding to particular sectors. Or, a rapid increase in funds to the sector could be followed by an equally rapid decline at a later date (Cassels: 39).

Defining a sustainable financial framework does not mean shying away from supporting increases in public funding and budget deficits where they are justified by well-designed programs that address key policy issues over a longer term. Private financing should be emphasized. Developing a sustainable financial framework involves setting priorities for both public and private financing of the sector.

BUILDING A MEDIUM-TERM EXPENDITURE PROGRAM FOR THE SECTOR

Once a feasible and appropriate aggregate level of allocations to the sector has been agreed on, the next step is to ensure correct allocations within the sector. The task is to make expenditures consistent with sectoral strategies and priorities, and to ensure that available sectoral resources are used as cost-effectively as possible (Cassels: 39). The underlying assumption is that greater impact will be achieved by (a) combining all donor and government resources in one program, and (b) focusing these integrated resources on priority interventions.

As stated above for the policy framework, an essential step in ensuring consistent allocations is for stakeholders to agree on the sector expenditure program. This stakeholder participation has to be structured to focus on priorities within overall resource constraints. Levels of government that will be included in implementation should be involved in stakeholder participation (Jones: 40). These lessons were underscored in the development of the Ethiopia education program. Initial attempts at consultation with regional officials placed no financial limits on suggestions, which then ballooned to unrealistic proportions. A second attempt set budgetary ceilings and the resulting

feedback was highly useful in setting and revising priorities.

Sector programs have to be explicit about resource allocation priorities (Peters and Chao: 182). Just as development of the sector policy is an ongoing process, so too is elaboration of the financial framework. Monitoring of actual expenditures must be done periodically in relation to planned allocations. This is essential to ensure full funding of priorities and to limit the scope for fungability. Monitoring, in turn, requires complete, up-to-date and readily available (i.e., transparent) information about actual expenditures. In addition, procedures must be in place for the appraisal of capital projects to provide a sound basis for annual budget negotiations (Cassels: 40).

Experiences thus far indicate that completely transparent information has been problematic. In Ethiopia the government officials announced plans to change intrasectoral budget priorities (increasing allocations to higher education, which was considered by donors to be of lower priority) just weeks after annual consultations with donors in which no allusion was made to the imminent changes. In several other cases, such as Ghana health and Zambia health, annual reviews were delayed or hampered by lack of timely information about actual expenditures.

Most disagreements in the preparation of sectoral expenditure programs have concerned (1) the relative balance between subsectors (tertiary health and education generally occupying a higher place in the set of priorities of government than of donors), and (2) the relative priority given to capital development vs. recurrent spending. In development of the Ethiopia health program substantial discussion took place on this topic that eventually achieved a better balance between capital and recurrent spending, one that was more feasible in the long run. Similar discussions took place during the development of the Ghana health program.

Another issue in long-term financial planning pertains to uncertainties about donor contributions. Donor commitment cycles are often out of phase with government budget cycles. Donors may not be able to commit funding at the time it is needed by government. Or, worse, they may commit funds, then not disburse. This happened for both the Ethiopia education and health programs. Several donors suspended assistance in response to the start of the war with Eritrea. The Mozambique education program addressed the problem of late donor commitments by financing a core program that can be expanded later as additional donors contribute.

Despite the importance of a careful review of investment programs and projects the sector-wide cases examined did not present much evidence of attention to government procedures for selection of investment subprojects. This contrasts with earlier sector investment projects, which focused on appraisal and selection of subprojects by an intermediary. (See Thomas (1994) and Johanson (1985).)

The level of financial analysis was weak in some of the cases reviewed. The Mozambique education program deferred the analysis of education finance until implementation. Zambia education deferred the sector expenditure review, making it a condition for phase II of the APL. It is difficult to see how intersectoral allocations and overall spending priorities can be made in the absence of thorough public expenditure reviews.

Finally, one case was observed of "best practice." Development of The Gambia education program used a computer-based projection model to assess the cost implications of alternative strategic choices based on core assumptions. This served two purposes: the model facilitated the selection of strategic alternatives, and it also became the basis for monitoring progress during implementation.

CHAPTER 6

DESIGNING IMPLEMENTATION SYSTEMS

In 1998 Utz (13-15) found that sector-wide programs in the Africa region suffered from 65% disbursement lags and registered 43% as problem projects (compared with an average of just 24% for all projects in the region.) In part these delays reflect the complexity of sector programs. Sector programs inherently are more complex than traditional projects, and being sector-wide, have to deal with the problems of the entire sector. Sector-wide programs also tend to be launched in the context of major institutional reforms such as restructuring of central ministries and devolution of authority to the field. The difficulty of these reforms tends to be underestimated. Another reason explaining weak implementation performance is weak institutional capacity of the recipient country (Cassels: 41). Utz (10) concluded that not enough attention was paid to implementation issues in the preparation of sector-wide programs.

Requirements for implementation should be regarded as high priority in the design of sector-wide approaches. The design of effective implementation systems involves four aspects: (a) analyzing existing institutional capacity and planning for its strengthening, (b) developing performance monitoring systems, (c) financial management, and (d) procurement. Each of these topics is treated in sequence below.

ANALYZING INSTITUTIONAL CAPACITY

Institutional capacity is complex and involves at least three types of capacity: (1) leadership capacity, (2) management of sectoral services, and (3) program management, including management of financial flows and procurement (Harrold: 22; Cassels: 41). In Chapter 1 a "Catch-22" was noted, i.e., the inherent tension between requiring good implementation capacity as a precondition for starting the development of a sector program and using the sector program to develop this capacity. Clearly an assessment of institutional capacity is needed to establish whether minimum levels of capacity exist both to start the process of program development and to decide whether implementation capacity warrants the committing of funds to the program. Several sources (Okidegbe: 17; Jones: 41) recommend starting with an assessment of institutional capacity and having an appropriate institutional framework in place before embarking on implementation. Harrold (26) refers to a sector institution assessment (SIA) as a critical means to form a judgment on government implementation.

Assessment of institutional capacity should concentrate on the key issues of incentives, accountability, workload, and control of access to resources (Harrold: 26). The Tanzania integrated roads program exemplifies why incentives are so important. Ultimately the program faltered because of a lack of these incentives for key implementation personnel. Road engineers in Tanzania were not paid well enough to carry out their additional duties assiduously under the program, and local contractors could not be paid fast enough to keep them working.

Analysis of institutional capacity should go beyond the limits of the sector organization. In particular, the analysis should consider the flow of funds.

This is made more important by the frequent use of sector programs to implement devolution of administrative authority from centralized systems to regional and district authorities. Constraints on the flow of funds is a common reason for under-disbursement in sector programs. Funds were allocated to regions in the Zambia health program, but did not get passed on to the intended districts. Initial disbursements have been slow under the Ethiopia education program in part because of difficulties in getting funds from the center to the regions. Analysis should also examine likely staff reactions to decentralization. In the Senegal health program resistance is being experienced to decentralization from several quarters. Institutional analysis could have pinpointed these likely points of resistance in advance so that compensatory measures could have been adopted.

Staff working on several of the programs reviewed felt that there had been insufficient analysis of institutional capacity prior to commitment of funds. These include Zambia education, Ethiopia education, and Zambia health. The Gambia education case stands out in contrast as an excellent example of systematic institutional analysis, as shown in Box 6.1.

Unfortunately, this type of institutional analysis is not cheap, in the order of approximately $50,000. One clear conclusion from the review is that institutional analysis is an essential prerequisite for commitment of funds under a sector program. Available tools for institutional analysis should be applied more systematically.

A well-designed Adaptable Program Loan (APL) can deal with institutional constraints. "Triggers" for future phases, for example, could be specific improvements in structure, staffing, or procedures under the first phase.

MONITORING PERFORMANCE

Proper monitoring of performance against agreements includes two things: (a) information systems

---

BOX 6.1

Institutional Analysis in The Gambia Education Program: An Example of Best Practice

One of the unique characteristics of the Gambia education APL is the systematic evaluation that was done of institutional capacity. This followed a methodology that analyzed all the proposed activities in the Program in terms of five criteria: whether (a) the functions and activities have an appropriate organizational home; (b) the level of leadership and management is effective; (c) sufficient operating funds are available for the implementation of assigned activities; (d) the unit has the right number of people with the right mix of skills—based on a workload analysis; and (e) key work practices are efficient and effective. This assessment identified several capacity gaps. For example, the analysis found that curriculum development and in-service teacher training had improper management responsibility outside the Ministry of Education. Another example, in terms of work practices, was the weak coordination among units in the Ministry. The next step was to consider alternatives to fill the capacity gap through (i) changed practices and procedures, (ii) spreading activities over a longer time—including the introduction of a two-phase approach and postponement of some activities to the second phase; (iii) reallocating financial and human resources; and (iv) reducing the scope of the development objectives. In the end the Gambia education APL included a detailed analysis of all major institutional components involved in the overall program and detailed capacity building measures.

Source: Gambia education case study.

to collect, analyze, and report data on implementation; and (b) procedures for joint review of performance. Each is presented in turn below.

Information Systems

Given the orientation of sector-wide improvements to processes (e.g., tracking improvements over time), the quality and timeliness of data collection are of paramount importance. Information on performance is doubly important in cases in which disbursements are made against achievements, as is the case in the Ghana health program. According to Cassels (43) and Peters and Chao (195) three types of data need to be collected: (a) monitoring of individual delivery centers and performance at various levels of the system against objectives, (b) aggregating performance for the sector as a whole against each objective, and (c) on processes such as policy development, institutional development, and management performance. The key attributes of performance indicators are clarity, consistency, specificity, sensitivity, and ease of collection (Harrold: 38). Moreover, the number of indicators should be kept to a manageable number. Donors should agree not to file any additional requests with the government for information, but live within agreed indicators.

The development of information systems involves several issues. Ideally, indicators should establish the extent to which growth of output can be attributed to better policies, efficiency gains in the administration of public expenditures, or improved delivery of goods and services (Okidegbe: 6). In practice, however, there are difficulties of measuring and especially attributing impact at the sectoral level (Grindle: 5). Moreover, establishment of systems for assessing impact takes time and requirements are consistently underestimated. So far, the development of data systems has received some attention, but remains weak in the development of sector programs (Jones: 30, 37, 41). Weaknesses of monitoring and evaluation have been identified by the Department for International Development (DFID) as the most

fundamental threat to the sustainability of the sector-wide approach. (Grindle: 5)

Experience from the implementation of Bank-funded sector programs shows that considerable time is indeed required to design and implement monitoring and evaluation schemes. The Zambia Agriculture SIP demonstrated this point. Virtually every sector program has suffered in the first two years from inadequate and late information needed to ascertain levels of performance. One practice to counter this phenomenon and ensure the reliability of the information is to use external agencies to collect or verify data, as is being done under the Pakistan Social Action Program and the Ghana health program (Harrold: 38). Some projects muddy the waters by having too many indicators, so that priorities get lost in the many types of data to be collected and reported. Referring to health programs, Peters and Chao (185) found there were 9 national level indicators in Senegal, 20 in Ghana, 23 in Mozambique, and 40 in Sierra Leone. The importance of indicators was underscored in the Zambia health program, which ran into difficulties when disagreements arose about the directions of policy change. Agreed, objectively verifiable, and explicit core indicators were missing. Without these it was difficult to ascertain whether the government was in compliance, as shown in Box 6.2.

Another particular issue about indicators arose in the Ethiopia education program. Final targets were clearly specified, but they had not been broken into interim steps for monitoring annual performance. Finally, indicators by themselves are not enough. As emphasized in the Ghana case, there must be a system to collect the information, analyze the results and report them.

Joint Reviews

Joint reviews between donors and government authorities are the main instrument for assessing progress, resolving issues, and reaching agreements on the program. The joint reviews are at the heart of sector-wide processes. In most cases they take the place of, or largely replace, supervision missions by

---

BOX 6.2
Lack of Monitoring Indicators in the Zambia Health Program

In hindsight, four years after the start of project implementation, it is clear that the directions for development of the sector were not made fully explicit. There were no objectively verifiable indicators that could define adherence or deviation from the agreed plan. Too much was left to interpretation and opinion. The Bank did not agree with the Government and other donor partners on outcome indicators, indicative targets, and milestones for jointly monitoring the program. In retrospect, useful indicators would have been spending as a proportion of budgets on primary, secondary, and tertiary facilities; and availability of drugs. There should have been specific, clearly stated milestones, e.g., the Central Board of Health (CBOH) established with an acceptable memorandum of understanding between CBOH and the Ministry of Health; legislation supporting decentralization passed, etc. It is therefore advisable first to get baseline data and agree on indicators and not to make commitments until there is explicit agreement on what constitutes progress.

Source: Zambia health case study.

---

donor agencies. Legal conditions are frequently tied to the processes, such as annual reporting, and financing of agreed annual plans (see Box 6.3, Senegal health).

These joint reviews normally take place twice a year, in late spring and fall. The spring meeting concerns actual progress over the past year and achievement of targets and objectives. The fall meeting deals with the establishment of targets and commitment of funds for the coming year. These meetings, and the information to be considered, need to be planned carefully in advance (Ghana health). According to supervision reports on sector-wide programs (Ethiopia health and education); (Senegal health, and Zambia education) the effectiveness of the joint reviews are often handicapped by weak government reporting on performance. In Zambia, the fall meetings were generally more successful than the spring meetings, partly because of the priority attached to commitment of funds for the following year.

Joint meetings serve the indispensable function of providing a venue for dealing with problems. A key question that those considering entering into sector programs should ask is: how will the partnership hold up over repeated conflicts and changes in

regime (Peters and Chao: 186, 190). The critical issue is not that difficulties will arise, but rather whether mechanisms and procedures are in place for dealing with them when they do (Cassels: 3). All parties must be prepared for negotiations and compromise in solving operational problems, characteristics that have not been typical of the larger donor agencies. Cassels wrote (56) that in handling disagreements it is helpful to classify potential problems according to the following hierarchy: (a) agreements on sector strategies and exclusion of activities inconsistent with sector programs, (b) degree of fit between policies and spending plans, (c) common management agreements, and (d) performance not up to expectations, e.g., funding shortfalls that should trigger formal consultation.

More thought and planning needs to be devoted to contingencies before commitment of funds (Jones: 37). Because of the wide scope, sector programs are more vulnerable to macroeconomic shocks than more narrow projects. Disruptions are probable. Staff turnover is so critical and likely that one reviewer said it could be "considered generic rather than incidental" (Jespersen: 4). In the Zambia health program major problems arose when a new Minister of

BOX 6.3
Modus Operandi for Senegal Health

The Sectoral Investment Program emphasizes a continuing policy dialogue and phased funding, based on yearly operational plans, eligibility criteria for program resources, and sector-wide performance indicators. This is achieved through joint Government/Donors annual implementation reviews. The joint annual reviews are the key element in the implementation process. The program is being implemented through a series of joint annual agreements based on an assessment of previous years' performance and operational plans and budgets based on priorities and established eligibility criteria for access to program funding. This procedure allows Government, IDA, and other financing institutions to adjust to changing conditions and performance, thereby building in a higher level of flexibility that will allow for more realistic planning on a year-by-year basis. Plans call for five such annual agreements, each covering one fiscal year from 1998 to 2002. Each will summarize the detailed individual agreement for specific categories of expenditure. Annual reviews are timed to coincide with the Government's fiscal year. Monitoring and information systems, common for all donors, are a key to the success of annual reviews. Two sets of data are collected: (a) critical performance benchmarks—for the first two years these include placement of program management staff, acceptable allocations to each expenditure category, levels of disbursement, recruitment and training of staff and Management Information Systems (MIS) in place in all districts; and (b) performance indicators for districts include: increases in the use of health facilities, proportion of children vaccinated, increases in pre-natal consultations and increases in contraceptive prevalence.

Source: Senegal health case study.

Health took over with a markedly different set of policies and priorities. Planning for contingencies such as these should be an integral part of good program preparation.

Providing Adequate Resources for Monitoring Implementation

Sector programs have clear resource implications that may not be fully appreciated by Bank management. These programs are much more complex than standard operations. The attempts to work through government procedures, the need to harmonize with other donors, the wide scope of activities covered, and the reforms introduced (e.g., decentralization) all add layers of complexity to the operation. Donors have to be concerned about all policies in the

sector, top to bottom, wall to wall. Examples of this were personnel strikes in Senegal and Ghana. These activities could be ignored under a project, but must be addressed under a sector program. Implementation requires continued sector analysis and updating of the policy framework. Extensive preparations are required for semiannual joint review missions. All these things imply the need for appropriate and sufficient staff and budget during implementation. The resources can come from several sources, including funds included in the loans/credits, e.g., for field audits, studies, and evaluations. Much of the burden will also fall on the Bank's supervision budget, but these budgets for sector programs have tended not to be proportional to the wider scope of activities involved in a sector-wide program. They tend to be underbudgeted in terms of the size and complexity of the operations. The consequence is less intensive coverage of subprograms. Realistic estimates should be made in advance of resource requirements and the various sources should be identified.

FINANCIAL MANAGEMENT

Budgeting and Expenditures

Another distinguishing characteristic of sector-wide programs is the use of regular government structures, systems, and procedures. The overall objective is to strengthen government systems by using and improving them. None is more important than the system for budgeting and expenditures. Since achievement of sectoral objectives depends on effective use of government resources, sector programs must be tied to regular procedures for budgeting and planning. The intention is ultimately to disburse funds through normal government channels rather than using special-purpose accounts and separate channels. Better management of public expenditures and systems is a critical requirement if there is to be progress toward government ownership and budgetary support (Jespersen: 6).

A precondition for the use of government financial systems, of course, is donor confidence in the financing system and a track record of proven capabilities (Jones: 27). The first step toward use of government procedures is strengthening the structure of the public budget to monitor spending better (Peters and Chao: 184). This is not a simple process and may take years or even decades to achieve. One of the reasons that Ghana has gone the furthest in pooling donor funds (discussed below) is the confidence that donors have in the financial management system. This confidence, in turn, is the product of decades of sustained work on its improvement.

Donors can frustrate budgetary reform by (a) disbursing money without regard to the national budget, or (b) failing actually to provide the funds when agreed (EU:11-12).

One exemplary practice identified in this review is the financial incentives for good implementation performance built into the Ghana health program. Disbursements are contingent on the level of performance. Disbursements are set at $7 million per year, but can be adjusted up or down by 50% based on actual performance by the Ghanaian

---

BOX 6.4
Varying Disbursements According to Performance in Ghana Health

An IDA Credit for US$35 million provides a base amount of US$7 million per year. An interesting feature of the Credit is the possibility to vary annual disbursements in relation to performance. Conditions for baseline funding include (a) the Government meets its fiscal commitments to financing the Program of Work (POW), and (b) audits of the POW demonstrate adequate fiscal probity. (SAR: 18). If these conditions are not met, the Bank would decrease IDA amounts below the baseline. Flexibility also exists to increase the amounts disbursed based on three additional conditions: (a) capacity to implement the POW as measured by ability to spend according to POW plans; (b) an increasing gap between the budget and available grant funds, in which case IDA funds could be used to fill the gap; and (c) strong showing on the agreed set of sector performance indicators. In the future it is expected that financing will be explicitly linked to performance on agreed sector indicators (SAR: 18). Consistent with this flexibility, Schedule 1 of the Credit Agreement leaves US$30 million of $35 million, or 86%, unallocated.

Source: Ghana health case study.

BOX 6.5
Zambia Health: The Start of Pooling Donor Funding

The Zambia program pioneered the use of "basket funding," or pooling of donor contributions into a common account. The idea of financing against the government budget started with the proposed DANIDA grant funds to districts. Although this idea did not materialize during the design stage, donors supported the concept during implementation. Donor funds were pooled for district grants and made use of common accounting and reporting procedures developed with DANIDA assistance. Separate donor accounts were established at the center. Funds were released monthly and were commingled at the district level, i.e., donor origins could not be identified. The release of funds by the center was negotiated with all donors. Each donor had veto power.

Source: Zambia health case study.

authorities in meeting program targets, as explained in Box 6.4.

Pooling of Donor Funds

The ultimate objective is "basket funding", or pooling of donor resources with government funds—in effect, pure budgetary support. These funds would then be dispersed, used, and accounted for through normal government channels. Under pooling of donor resources different funds from different donors would no longer be identified separately, and would no longer be earmarked for different purposes. Payments would be made into and out of a common account rather than via reimbursement of specific expenditures (Cassels: 46). There are two steps toward this ultimate goal: (1) pooling of donor funds; and (2) commingling of pooled donor funds with government funds.

The potential benefits of pooled donor funds are enhanced government ownership of the program, incentives for better budget planning, less likelihood of budgetary imbalances, strengthening rather than bypassing government procedures, rapid disbursements, lower costs to manage donor funds, and greater opportunities for budgetary reforms (EU: 6).

The requirements for pooling on the recipient side are assurances that funds will be used as in-

tended, transparency, and accountability. Many donors are reluctant or unable to pool their funds with other donors. Some of the reasons apply to the donors themselves. Some donors simply do not have instruments for financing recurrent costs or providing direct budget support. Others find it difficult to adjust their financing procedures and timetables. Some do not want to lose the identity of their funds as a donor (i.e., attribution, or "raising the flag"). Other reasons apply to the recipient government. The budget process may be deficient, allowing diversion of funds from high to low priority items. Rivalries may block disbursement of funds to intended beneficiaries. It may not be possible to ensure full accounting of funds and the risks of wastage may be unacceptably high (EU: 7; Peters and Chao: 185; Jespersen: 10).

There are only a few examples of pooling of funds in sector-wide projects in the Bank. These include the Zambia technical assistance and health district funds (see Box 6.5), common disbursements under the Bangladesh health sector program; district funds under the Senegal health program; and preparation studies for the Zambia education program. The best example of pooling of funds is the Ghana health sector program, as described in Box 6.6.

In the Ghana Health program, the Bank accepted that it would not be able to trace the specific expen-

---

BOX 6.6
Pooling of Donor Funds in Ghana Health

A unique feature of the IDA Credit is the use of a common account and pooling of resources. The Ministry of Health has gone a long way to establish financial management systems that will ensure appropriate use and accounting of funds. The majority of donor funds, including the IDA Credit, will be managed on lines of existing government procedures. Some earmarked project funds will continue over the medium term, but the preferred donor financing system is an untied contribution into a common Health Account. Once IDA and other donor funds reach the Health Account, there is no further identification of the funds by donor origin, thus the funds are genuinely pooled. IDA is putting all its contributions to the program into the pool. Three other donors are putting part of their contributions into the pool. The rest of the resources and those of other donors are earmarked funds, but are not provided in the traditional manner, as they are planned according to the annual planning and budgeting cycle, and are channeled through the Financial Controller in an accountable manner, rather than directly to program managers in isolation of other funding. The Health Account funds are put into a bank account under the direct control of MOH and the Controller and Accountant General. These funds are then distributed to all eligible health units that meet minimum "Readiness Criteria", including: (1) submission of annual budget accompanied by quantified targets and objectives; (2) satisfactory procedures and collecting and accounting for independently generated funds; (3) adequate procedures for authorization of payments; (4) adequate and timely maintenance of accounts; and (5) adequate staff and procedures to prepare monthly reports on revenues and expenditures.

Source: Ghana health case study.

---

diture of Bank funds. Instead, it relies on annual audits of government expenditures, including pooled government, donor, and IDA funds.

Examples of pooling are clearly in the minority. Instead of pooling, most sector-wide programs thus far earmark funds (i.e., typing of donor funds to a specific activity output.) For example, parallel financing channels were specifically identified in the Zambia education program and these alternative channels helped greatly to clarify the choices for donors. (See Box 6.7). Even Basket funding in Ghana, Zambia health, and Senegal health operate in parallel with project accounts for individual donors (Grindle: 5).

As is pointed out in the Senegal health case, pooling of resources need not be the first step, but is the ultimate objective. There can be stages toward achieving full budgetary support (Jespersen: 10).

Lender of Last Resort

Considerable confusion surrounds this topic. It means the Bank, since it loans money, will finance what cannot be financed through grant funds (because generally it is better for a government to receive grant money than loans[1]). It means the Bank

---

[1] Still, it should be remembered that the grant element in IDA loans is almost 80% because of the low interest rate in relation to inflation.

will finance the residual left after grant funds have been allocated. However, it does not mean that low priority items should be financed. Jones (11) has pointed out the risk that the donor of last resort will end up financing items of lower priority or those that are less fashionable. However, being lender of last resort does not really mean financing lower priority items, because the expenditure program will have been thoroughly vetted to ensure that only important items are funded. In practice, it probably means the Bank will end up financing more civil works because other donors generally do not want to use their grant funds for building. Financing of civil works is not a problem if the budget has been properly screened and low priority components have been removed. It really does not matter who finances what, so long as the full program – limited to the highest priority activities – gets funded. As Harrold (35) pointed out, "Under the sector-wide approach the Bank's project is the sector, not the actual goods and services it happens to finance."

Application of the donor of last resort concept means different things depending on how program funds are managed. If funds are earmarked, then the donor of last resort finances those items of the program that are left after other grant donors select the components they wish to finance. When funds are pooled, all components and items are financed out of a common account. Under these circumstances the lender of last resort finances the gap between available (grant) funds and total resource requirements.

In practice, being lender of last resort requires the Bank to maintain flexibility to adjust the objects and amounts of its disbursements from year to year. Specifically, Bank sector programs need to keep large unallocated amounts in the schedule of disbursements. This is clearly seen in the Ethiopia education program that has about two thirds of the total funds unallocated.

A donor of last resort is also needed for a sector program because promised donor funds often do not

---

BOX 6.7

Multiple Channels for Donor Funding in Zambia Education

The Preparatory Fund for the Basic Education Sector Program received funds into a common account ("pooling") by several donors, including the United Kingdom, The Netherlands, Ireland and Norway. This became the model that Government wished to use for the full program implementation. "Pooling" was recognized as the ideal method during the joint appraisal, but was not foreseen as being acceptable to most donors because of weaknesses in existing capacity for financial management. Instead, the Program was explicitly designed to allow flexibility in the channeling of funds by donors. The following external financing modalities are recognized:

Source: Zambia education case study.

Category	Case 1	Case 2	Case 3	Case 4
Funds controlled by:	MOE	MOE	MOE	Donor
Funds available for which Program components:	All	All	Limited number	One or a small number
"Pooling" of funds in common account	Yes	No	No	No
Examples of donors using each method	Dutch, Irish	IDA		

BOX 6.8
Financing of the ESSP in Mozambique

The financing plan for the program was drafted during the joint donor assessment mission in May 1998 and further refined during appraisal in late 1998. By appraisal a total of about US$85 million had been committed to ESSP by various donors to support ongoing activities that were part of the program. Approximately US$105 million in additional funds were expected to be provided by donors over the five-year program period. The schedule for agreement on new funds would follow the program cycles of the various agencies. The normal approval cycles for the various donors meant that commitment of new funding would be drawn out over two or three years. A number of donors also (e.g., Denmark, the Netherlands, Sweden, Ireland, and the United Kingdom/DfID) planned to provide about US$70 million of their funding for the program through direct budgetary support. Budget support was entirely new. No one knew exactly how to do it. Some donors complicated the funding picture further by making their new funding contingent on the provision of budgetary support by at least a core group of donors. Consequently, there was considerable uncertainty over when (and perhaps whether) new funding would materialize from several key donors. The Bank therefore shifted from its intended role as donor of last resort to the immediate financing of several core components. Financing of the core program by the Bank was designed to ensure continued financing of the program as a whole pending the release of other donor funding.

Source: Mozambique education case study.

materialize when needed. The Mozambique education program financed a core program to which other donor funds could be added when ready, as explained in Box 6.8.

In practice, the Bank as lender of last resort has had mixed success. In the Ethiopia education program it helped allay suspicions by other donors that the Bank was trying to dominate, but complications arose when other donors delayed in providing funds. In Zambia health, the Bank's special account ended up being used as a slush fund to finance anything not provided elsewhere. This underscores the importance of agreement in advance on an exclusive expenditure program.

The important thing, in the final analysis, is that (a) program formulation and expenditure reviews have eliminated unjustifiable expenditures, and (b) there is explicit agreement in advance of what is excluded from the expenditure program. Moreover, the "patchwork" approach—where donors pick and

choose components they wish to finance, with the Bank picking up the remainder—should be accepted only as a step toward the broader strategy of pooling and channeling funds through the budget.

PROCUREMENT

Goods and Works: The harmonization of financial procedures seems almost simple by comparison to the difficulties in harmonizing different donor requirements on procurement. This is because the procurement rules of donors are often not designed for a sectoral approach (Jespersen: 10), but rather to stimulate the purchase of goods and services from the donor country. "Rules of origin" are thus a major obstacle, but waivers are reportedly possible in some cases (Cassels: 47). On the government side, the authority for procurement and capital projects can be so complicated as to stall the entire system.

There is a risk under harmonization that the Ministry is forced to adopt the procedures of the most restrictive donor (Cassels: 47). In most cases procurement is divided and follows the rules of the source of funds (Peters and Chao: 184), a practice that is viewed as sub-optimal by many. One problem mentioned was the lack of early involvement of financial and procurement specialists at the design stage of sector programs. Another problem was a discrepancy between a standard procurement schedule in the Credit Agreement of the Ghana health program and the intentions expressed in the project appraisal document (PAD) for common procurement procedures. (See the Ghana health case.)

Technical Assistance: More success has been achieved in establishing common funds for technical assistance. Examples include Zambia health and education; Pakistan SAP, Bangladesh health, and Zambia agriculture SIP (Okidegbe: 9). On another topic, Harrold stressed the value of minimizing external technical assistance and even included it as the sixth major characteristic of SIPs. In practice many donors have insisted on the use of external technical assistance, especially in financial management and procurement. There is general agreement that external technical assistance should (a) not be used in line positions; (b) be provided only in response to government requests; and (c) be used to complement, not supplant, local expertise (Harrold: 17; Jones: 27; Okidegbe: 9). If too much technical assistance is requested, this is symptomatic of deeper problems, such as disagreements on strategy or a poor institutional environment (Jones: 28). It may also stem from unrealistic expectations for the sector program and a tendency to encourage state-of-the-art where this is unrealistic (Jespersen: 11).

Finally, the staffing implications of sectoral programs need to be considered carefully. This means: (a) frequent interaction between government officials and donor staff who can speak authoritatively on behalf of donors – which may require staffing of local offices (Cassels: 58-59); (b) changing or upgrading of donor staff capacity to deal continuously with policy analysis and issues; and (c) adequate budgeting for supervision that tends to be 50-100% (Zambia 50%, Mozambique education 100%) greater than normal projects. Larger-than-normal budgets are fully justified by the scope of activities and subprograms, sometimes equivalent to several projects.

CHAPTER 7

MAIN FINDINGS AND RECOMMENDATIONS

Sector programs are inherently complex. Complexity is derived from: (a) the broad scope, the concern with everything in the sector—top to bottom, wall to wall—(b) donor coordination—never an easy task, but made even more complicated by the extremely high number of donors involved in many of the African countries, (c) the attempts to channel external resources through the government budget, and (d) the simultaneous efforts at major sectoral reforms, such as decentralization. All these factors add layers of complexity to sector programs. Complexity is not a weakness per se. It only becomes a weakness when ambition exceeds capacity.

Complexity comes at a price, in terms of more time and resources required for development and supervision of sector programs than traditional projects (in the order of 50%-100% more) and more time required for program development and implementation. The staffing implications are: (a) different mix of skills than for projects, with an emphasis on policy analysis and ability to negotiate with high level officials on policy matters; (b) the need for a local technical presence to keep the dialogue going and coordinate with other donors; and (c) possibly more frequent missions to keep abreast of sector developments.

BOX 7.1

Changes of Personnel and Policy Derail the Zambia Health Program

During program development and implementation there have been four different ministers of health. The second minister tried to sidetrack the reforms, but Parliamentarians supported the health manifesto and brought him back into line. Broad approval was required to delink the health staff from the civil service (including defeating lawsuits) create the Central Board of Health, and turn districts into autonomous boards. Thus, the reform had broad-based and high-level support. Prior experiences with changes of leadership had not altered the directions of reform. All that changed in 1998 when a new minister of health was appointed. The new minister changed priorities and placed emphasis on support for tertiary care institutions and centralization. This reversed some reform strategies. The new minister took an adversarial relationship with donors. The openness that had prevailed evaporated. The minister prevented an open dialogue in the 1998 annual meeting. Implementation of the program came to a standstill. DANIDA suspended most of its program. Few funds have been disbursed from the IDA Credit in over one year. Several procurement applications have been rejected by the Bank.

Source: Zambia health case study.

It is still too early to tell whether sector-wide approaches in the social sector are making an impact, but some of the successes and weaknesses to date can be identified, as follows:

SUCCESSES OF THE SECTOR-WIDE APPROACH

Sector-wide approaches address many of the problems and issues that contribute to poor performance by projects. They have strengthened the ability of the government to oversee the sector, develop policies and allocate resources. (Peters and Chao: 188). They have led to the development of comprehensive plans and strategies. In all the eight cases reviewed the government developed a long term vision and strategy for the sector. The dialogues conducted during program preparation have had success in eliminating imbalances between capital and recurrent spending. Sector programs have also been successful in achieving decentralized planning in several cases (e.g., Zambia health—bottom-up planning of district grants; Ethiopia education and health both achieved district plans and strengthened district planning capacities). Sector programs have forged strong links between policy development, allocation of funds, and performance monitoring (Peters and Chao: 184). As concluded in the Ghana health case study, "For the first time health policies are being explicitly linked to resource allocation in a comprehensive manner, covering all government and donor financing." Stakeholder consultation and participation has been strengthened (Jones: 14-15). All the eight cases were built on stakeholder consultation. Frameworks for donor coordination have been established. Some common procedures have been achieved, particularly on joint appraisal systems, annual reviews, and common reporting systems. Initial steps have been made in a few projects to move to budget support by pooling external resources and channeling them through the government budget. These measures have reduced the administrative burden of external assistance on recipient governments. Finally, sector programs have

succeeded in increasing the relative shares (and absolute amounts) of public resources going into the respective sectors.

WEAKNESSES

Design of Sector Programs

Some of the sector programs reviewed did not include rigorous sector analysis. Since policy analysis is an ongoing process, staff felt that any gaps could be made up during implementation. However, this risks an inappropriate or misguided policy package.

The main weakness identified in the preparation of sector-wide programs was the lack of systematic analysis of implementation capacity. Staff felt that more could have been done to analyze and fix implementation weaknesses. The tendency for overly ambitious sector programs in relation to existing capacities has been noted, a corollary of their complexity. Institutional analysis can be an antidote to overly ambitious tendencies.

The review underscores the importance of monitoring indicators. Several problems occurred. Explicit indicators were lacking by which to determine and demonstrate deviation from policy agreements (Zambia health). In another case, Ethiopia education, targets were not broken into annual indicators for assessing the rate of progress. Other programs have tended to include too many indicators.

Implementation of Sector Programs

Problems and difficulties were the norm rather than the exception during implementation. The problems can be categorized into three types: (a) Changes in the macroeconomic environment. The war between Ethiopia and Eritrea is just such a change in the environment that caused financing agreements with other donors to unravel. (b) Changes in policy directions. Ethiopia education may have changes in policy direction, as indicated by changes in budget priorities for higher education. Zambia health experienced major changes of policy that led to a de facto suspension of the program, as described in Box 7.1. (c) Changes in key personnel. The people who champion the sector program often are replaced by others less familiar with, and less committed to, the sector program. In the Zambia health and The Gambia education cases these personnel changes led to at least temporary delays in implementation.

Problems and changes are inevitable. This fact suggests the need for sensitivity and risk analysis as a basis for careful contingency planning. Yet, this does not appear to have been done in the cases reviewed. Bank staff may not appreciate the special risks involved in dealing with ambitious sector programs. None has apparently undertaken contingency planning in advance. One contingency for which the Zambian health program was unprepared was the complete breakdown in dialogue and de facto suspension of the program. The Bank had no remedies to apply except the extreme measures of formal suspension and cancellation of the program.

Problems were also experienced in setting up data collection systems for the key indicators. Almost all cases note weaknesses in management information and reporting systems (examples: Ethiopia education and health; Senegal health; Zambia education).

All sector programs expect a great deal from the joint review process, perhaps too much. Virtually all cases expressed disappointment with joint reviews. The capacity required for government to organize meaningful annual reviews has been underestimated. This includes (a) information retrieval on process, product, and impact, (b) conducting ongoing studies and analyses on specific issues, and (c) planning detailed budgets.

RECOMMENDATIONS FOR BEST PRACTICE

Based on the findings of the review the following points are recommended as best practice.

A. Meet the Preconditions for Starting

(1) Ensure that the prerequisites are met for entering into the development of a sector-wide approach. Do not undertake a sector-wide approach unless the client has (i) a modicum of stability, (ii) strong commitment to an integrated, collaborative process, and (iii) at least a minimum level of institutional capacity. In addition, ensure that the donor agency allocates adequate resources and the right profile of staff for developing a sector program.

B. Establish a Collaborative Process

(1) Do not rush the process of policy development. Sector approaches are a long haul, not a quick fix. Time must be allowed for reaching agreements on policy issues and interventions, appropriate procedures, legislation and clear delineation of responsibilities to ensure sustainability (Jespersen: 12).

(2) Recognize that success ultimately depends on the level of trust among partners. Trust, in turn, is based on openness, transparency, negotiation, and compromise. Appropriate mechanisms must be in place by which all parties can raise and address problems and their concerns.

(3) Spell out the rights and responsibilities of all parties on paper at the start in a Statement of Intent, and later in a Memorandum of Understanding (or Credit Agreement) and Code of Practice.

(4) Follow Government's lead, but ensure that the ownership and participation is increased progressively from a narrow group of reformers and includes participation of central ministries and legislatures.

(5) Harmonize procedures that are feasible immediately, such as reporting, joint reviews, and monitoring systems. Also start

with immediate steps to strengthen and improve government systems. Get central agencies to work on generic systems for all sectors, such as finance and procurement, rather than repeating the work sector by sector.

(6) Define the role of a donor lead agency in advance to avoid misunderstandings. Provide sufficient administrative funds to pay for the high costs of coordination.

(7) Establish a joint technical assistance fund for project preparation to start the pooling of resources on a small scale.

C. Establish a Comprehensive Policy Framework

(1) Start with a comprehensive policy framework covering the sector as a whole even if subsequent investment programs have to be limited to particular subsectors because of capacity limitations.

(2) Help build stronger analytical underpinnings for sector-wide programs by improving the quality and rigor of sector analysis during initial program design.

(3) Recognize that policy analysis is an important ongoing function during program execution and focus attention (i) on building local capacity for continuing policy analysis during implementation, and (ii) on building better information systems for data collection.

(4) Continue the good work shown on stakeholder consultation. Widen the consultations beyond the bureaucracy to include front-line service workers and beneficiaries. Use a clearly defined resource envelope to ensure realism and facilitate hard choices among competing priorities.

(5) Have explicit policy agreement on basic principles and priorities before loan approval, an explicit list of policies on which consensus has not yet been reached, and a process for reaching consensus through further study and dialogue. Use an adaptable program loan (APL) with "triggers" set for achieving consensus on difficult areas of policy.

D. Develop Financial Parameters

(1) If it is not possible to invest in the sector as a whole, nonetheless monitor expenditures sector-wide to ensure reasonable intrasectoral allocations.

(2) Conduct public expenditure reviews before commitment of funds to establish an overall resource envelope for the sector. Do not defer this to the implementation phase.

(3) Use budget ceilings to force better selection of priorities, as when regions prepare sectoral programs.

(4) Devote attention to the establishment of sound government criteria and procedures for appraisal and selection of specific investment projects.

(5) Meticulously plan the flow of funds from the center to regions and districts to avoid the typical delays in disbursements.

(6) Where other donor funding is uncertain establish a core program of donor assistance with Bank financing, and add to the core as additional financing materializes.

(7) Use computer models for expenditure projections during preparation and use the same models during implementation for monitoring performance.

(8) Spell out the role of the lender of last resort. In particular, agree in advance on what specifically is excluded from the expenditure plan.

(9) Accept "patchwork" arrangements—where donors earmark funds for particular components—only as a step toward the optimal strategy, which is the pooling and channeling of donor funds through normal government budgets.

E. Build Management Systems and Capacity

(1) Use existing techniques more systematically and rigorously for institutional analysis to identify and address weaknesses and constraints before embarking on a sector program. Go beyond organizational analysis to consider staff incentives, identify who stands to gain and lose from program implementation and plan in detail the flow of funds to beneficiaries. Since institutional analysis is costly, budget the requirements separately and fully in project preparation. Consider using an APL to overcome structural constraints for later phases.

(2) Focus early and sharply on the development of monitoring and evaluation systems. Limit the number of indicators to priorities and ensure that they indicate clearly whether the program is on track annually.

(3) Design joint review procedures in advance and ensure that workable mechanisms are in place to identify, address, and resolve problems. Build government capacity to manage joint reviews.

(4) Involve financial and procurement specialists early in the design phase to help in developing appropriate systems.

(5) Link disbursements to achievements to provide incentives for good performance.

(6) Engage in better risk analysis and contingency planning for various types of occurrences. Think through systematically what would happen if critical changes happened in the macro-environment, e.g., (a) if macroeconomic shocks reduced sectoral allocations below planned targets; (b) if disagreements arose on the policy framework; and (c) if key staff changed. Devise a set of courses of action for each contingency. For example, assuming that key personnel inevitably will change, (i) broaden the participation of stakeholders, (ii) provide continuous training and briefings for new personnel involved, (iii) involve higher levels in the approval process, e.g., cabinets, and (iv) root the programs in legislation. Devise and install remedies at the design stage in case things do not work out and the program deviates markedly from the plan.

(7) After tapping other sources for financing studies and reviews, be prepared to finance substantially larger than normal budget coefficients for the supervision of sector programs, recognizing that ongoing analytical work is costly to review and the scope of sector-wide programs encompasses the equivalent of multiple projects.

The net effect of the above recommendations is to expand the list of things that must be done before loan or credit approval, making the preparation process even more demanding for a development program than a traditional project. In summary, the following steps should be considered as *essential prerequisites for commitment of funding* (i. e., in place by time of Board presentation) for sector-wide operations:

(a) *Policy framework developed*, based on rigorous sector analysis, including specific three-year work program (Ethiopia education).

(b) Wide *consultations with stakeholders* and donors have been held, and agreement reached on priorities.

(c) *Public expenditure review* or social sector expenditure review completed; overall *financial parameters defined* in terms of targeted intersectoral allocations and a *budget envelope* for the sector, and agreement on *budget priorities* for the first two years (Ethiopia health).

(d) *Institutional capacity analysis* completed and agreement reached on early implementation of a program to fill identified gaps.

(e) *Monitoring indicators identified* that show clearly whether program implementation is on track; *data collection system designed* and in place on processes, system delivery and impact (Ghana health).

(f) The modus operandi designed for *joint reviews and problem resolution*, i.e., mechanisms for common reporting, joint annual reviews of progress, budget planning, discussion differences).

(g) The role of *donor of last resort clearly spelled out* (and specifically what is excluded from the agreed expenditure program), and a staged *plan to achieve pooling* of resources among donors.

(h) Risk analysis prepared as a basis for *detailed contingency planning* for changes in (a) the macro-environment; (b) the policy framework; and (c) key staff. As part of the contingency planning, remedies should have been defined for noncompliance with, or substantial deviations from, agreements.

(i) Provision of the *correct profile of staff and adequate resources* (including outside financing and internal budgets) for program supervision.

The following are other *desirable but not essential conditions* for commitment of funds:

(a) Donor agreements reached on pooling of resources.

(b) Financial incentives included for good performance.

(c) Harmonization of procedures for financial management and procurement (likely to be a medium to long term goal.)

Bibliography

General

European Union. 1997. "Establishing an Education Sector Development Programme." EU Horizon 2000 Meeting of Education Experts of the Commission and Member States, Brussels, 10-11 November, 1997.

Gould, Jeremy, T. Takala, and Marko Nokkala. 1998. "How Sectoral Programs Work: An Analysis of Education and Agriculture Sector Programs in Zambia, Ethiopia, Mozambique and Nepal." Institute of Development Studies, University of Helsinki, presented to the DAC 1999 Annual Meeting, DAC Informal Network on Institutional and Capacity Development (I/CD), May 3-5, 1999 Ottawa Canada.

Johanson, Richard. 1995. "Sector Lending in Education." World Bank. December.

Okidegbe, Nwanze. 1997. "Fostering Sustainable Development: The Sector Investment Program." World Bank Discussion Paper No. 363.

Orbach, Eliezer. 1999. "How to Assess the Capacity of a Client Government to Implement an Education Development Project." World Bank.

Oxfam. 1999. "Education Now: Break the Cycle of Poverty."

Thomas, Chris. 1994. "Education Lending Instruments." World Bank.

UNICEF, 1999. "Overview Paper on Challenges to Promoting Basic Education for All Through Sectoral Approaches in Education." Eva Jespersen, draft, February 19.

World Bank. 1998. *Assessing Aid: What Works, What Doesn't and Why.* World Bank Policy Research Report. Oxford University Press.

Africa Regional

Donors to African Education. 1993. "Issues in the Implementation of Education Sector Programs and Projects in Sub-Saharan Africa." DAE Task Force Meetings, October.

Grindle, John. 1999. "Donor Harmonization in Sector Programmes: Issues and Challenges." PROAGRI High Level Meeting, Dublin. March 29.

Harrold, Peter, and Associates. 1995. "The Broad Sector Approach to Investment Lending." World Bank Discussion Papers: Africa Technical Department Series, No. 302. Washington, D.C.

Jones, Stephen P. 1997. "Sector Investment Programs in Africa: Issues and Experience," World Bank Technical Paper No. 374.

Sawyerr, Harry. 1997. "Country-Led Aid Coordination in Ghana." Association for the Development of Education in Africa. Paris.

Utz, Robert. 1998. "Sector Investment Programs in the Africa Region: A Review." World Bank. June 26.

THE EDUCATION SECTOR

General

Ratchille Macrae Associates. 1999. "Sector-Wide Approaches to Education: A Strategic Analysis." Study funded by the U.K. Department for International Development (DFID). June.

UNICEF. 1999. The State of the World's Education: 1999. New York.

Watkins, Kevin. 1999. "Education Now: Break the Cycle of Poverty." Oxfam International, U.K.

Africa

Rakotomanana, Michel, et al. 1998. "Sector-Wide Approaches (SWAPs) and Donor Coordination in Educational Development in Africa: Perspectives for Enhancing Japan's Participation." Japan International Cooperation Agency, USA Office. May 30.

Verspoor, Adriaan. 1999. "Knowledge and Finance for Education in Africa." Draft, World Bank, September.

Ethiopia

Martin, John, and Riitta Oksanen, and Tuomas Takala.1999. "Preparation of the Education Sector Development Programme in Ethiopia: Reflections by Participants." Cambridge Education Consultants, UK and FTP International, Finland. Final Report, 7 June 1999.

World Bank. 1998. "Program Appraisal Document on a Proposed International Development Association Credit in the Amount of US$100 Million Equivalent to the Federal Democratic Republic of Ethiopia for the Education Sector Development Program." Human Development IV and Country Department 6, Africa Region, Report No. 17739-ET, May 4, 1998.

World Bank. 1999. "Quality at Entry Assessment: Guidance Questionnaire" as part of the Quality At Entry Report for CY 1998, on the Ethiopia Education Sector Development Program. (Communicated by Dora Aku Adoteye to Prem Garg, EM 10/8/99.)

The Gambia

World Bank. 1998. "Project Appraisal Document on a Proposed Credit in the Amount of SDR 15.0 Million to the Republic of The Gambia for a Third Education Sector Project in the Support of the First Phase of the Third Education Sector Program," Human Development II, Country Department 14, Report No. 17903-GM, August 7, 1998.

Guinea

World Bank. 1990. "Report and Recommendation of the President of the International Development Association to the Executive Directors on a Proposed Credit of SDR 15.4 Million to the Republic of Guinea for an Education Sector Adjustment Credit." Report No. P-5288-GUI, May 11, 1990.

World Bank. 1995. "Implementation Completion Report: Republic of Guinea, Education Sector Adjustment Credit (Credit 2155-GUI)," Population and Human Resources Division, Western Africa Department, Africa Region, Report No. 14617, June 16, 1995.

World Bank. 1995. "Staff Appraisal Report, Republic of Guinea: Equity and School Improvement Project." Population and Human Resources Operations Division, Western Africa Department, Report No. 13472-GUI, April 7, 1995.

Lesotho

World Bank. 1999. "Project Appraisal Document on a Proposed Credit in the Amount of SDR 15 Million to the Kingdom of Lesotho for a Second Education Sector Development Project in Support of the First Phase of the Education Sector Program." Human Development 1, Country Department 1, Africa Region, Report No. 18388-LSO, March 25, 1999.

Mozambique

Republica de Mocambique. 1998. "Education Sector Strategic Plan: 1997-2001: Reviving Schools and Expanding Opportunities." Ministry of Education, Maputo, April 1998.

World Bank.1999. "Project Appraisal Document on a Proposed Credit in the Amount of 51.1 Million SDR (US$ 71 Million Equivalent) to the Republic of Mozambique for an Education Sector Strategic Program (ESSP)." Human Development 1, Country Department 2, Africa Region, Report No. 18681-MOZ, January 22, 1999.

Zambia

Chilangwa, Barbara Y. 1999. "Issues, Experiences, Challenges and Lessons in the Process of Establishing the Zambian Basic Education Sub-Sector Investment Programme (BESSIP)." Paper prepared for the annual meeting of the DAC's Institutional and Capacity Development Network, Ottawa, Canada, May 3-5, 1999.

World Bank. 1999. "Program Appraisal Document on a Proposed Credit in the Amount of SDR 28.5 Million to the Republic of Zambia in Support of the First Phase of the Basic Education Subsector Investment Program (BESSIP)." Human Development 1, Country Department 2, Africa Region, Report No. 19008 ZA, March 5, 1999.

THE HEALTH SECTOR

Cassels, Andrew. 1997. "A Guide to Sector-Wide Approaches for Health Development: Concepts, Issues and Working Arrangements." WHO, DANIDA, DFID and EU.

European Union. 1999. "Sector-Wide Approaches (SWAPs) as a Means to Develop Sustainable Health Services and Policies." Health Experts Meeting, January 1999.

Ethiopia

World Bank. 1998. *Development Credit Agreement:*

Health Sector Development Program Support Project. Credit Number 3140 ET. October 30.

World Bank. 1998. "Program Appraisal Document on a Proposed Credit in the Amount of SDR 75.1 million (US$100 Million Equivalent) to the Federal Democratic Republic of Ethiopia for a Health Sector Development Program." Report No. 18366-ET. September 24.

Ghana

Annan, Joe. 1999. "Ghana Health Sector-wide Programme: A Case Study." JSA Consultants, Ltd., Accra. Prepared for DAC I/CD Network and Policy Branch of CIDA, April 1999.

Decaillet, Francois. 1999. "Ghana: Health Sector Support Project—Back to Office Report." June 1, 1999.

Peters, David, and Shiyan Chao. 1998. "The Sector-Wide Approach in Health: What Is It? Where Is It Leading?" *International Journal of Health Planning and Management* 13: 177-190.

Republic of Ghana. 1998. "Memorandum of Understanding: Ghana Health Sector Programme of Work." April 30.

Republic of Ghana. 1999. "Health Sector 5-Year Programme of Work 1997-2001: 1998 Review." Ministry of Health, Accra, April.

World Bank. 1997. "Memorandum and Recommendation of the President of the International Development Association to the Executive Directors on a Proposed Credit in the Amount Equivalent to SDR 25.1 Million to the Republic of Ghana for a Health Sector Program Support Project." Report No. P 7179 GH, September 25, 1997.

World Bank. 1997. "Staff Appraisal Report: Republic of Ghana Health Sector Support Program." Human Development III, Ghana Country Department, Report No. 16467-GH, September 25, 1997.

"Aide Memoire: Joint Ministry of Health—Health Partners Summit Meeting (May 5-7, 1999), Review of the 1998 Programme of Work." 7 May 1999.

Senegal

World Bank. 1997. "Staff Appraisal Report: Republic of Senegal, Integrated Health Sector Development Program." Report No. 16756-SE. August 8.

Zambia

Joint Donor and Ministry of Health Statements. 1994, 1995, 1996, 1997.

Mahler, Halfdan, et al. 1997. "Comprehensive Review of the Zambian Health Reforms." Report of an independent review in September 1996. May 1997.

McLaughlin, Julie. 1997. "What Can We Learn from Implementation of a Sector-Wide Investment Approach to Lending?" Presentation at HNP Training Day for HD Resident Mission Staff. 19 March.

———. 1998. "Supervision Report: Zambia Health Mission". April 2.

Republic of Zambia Ministry of Health. 1998. "Memorandum of Understanding Between the Ministry of Health and Cooperating Partners in the Health Sector." July.

World Bank. No date. "Turning the Tables for Zambia's Health System." Handout in the "Investing in People" and "The World Bank in Action." Human Development Department.

World Bank. 1994. "Staff Appraisal Report, Zambia: Health Sector Support Project." Human Resources Division, Southern Africa Department, Report No. 13480-ZA. October 14, 1999.

List of World Bank Staff Interviewed

1. Arvil Van Adams (Ethiopia education)
2. Anwar Bach-Baouab (Senegal health)
3. Rosemary Bellew (The Gambia education)
4. David Berk (Ethiopia health)
5. Nicholas Burnett
6. Francois Decaillet (Ghana health)
7. Linda Dove
8. Birger Fredriksen
9. Donald Hamilton (Mozambique education)
10. Bruce Jones (Zambia education)
11. Julie McLaughlin (Zambia health)
12. Paud Murphy (Zambia education)
13. Eliezer Orbach (The Gambia education)
14. Ok Pannenborg
15. Robert Prouty (Guinea education Secal)
16. Jee-Peng Tan
17. Adriaan Verspoor
18. Steve Weissman

Ethiopia Health Case Study[1]
Health Sector Development Program Support Project

BACKGROUND

Ethiopia's burden of disease is dominated by acute respiratory infection and peri-natal and maternal conditions, followed by malaria, nutritional deficiency, diarrhea, and AIDS. The top 10 causes of mortality account for 74 percent of all deaths and 81 percent of discounted life years (DLYs) lost prematurely. The main issues in the health sector are: (1) low and inequitable coverage of basic health services (only about 45 percent of the population has access to a health facility); (2) low quality of services because of lack of drugs, poorly trained staff, and poor personnel management and supervision; (3) inefficiency in the use of resources in terms of concentration of available resources in urban areas and skewed allocations toward curative care. Historically the health sector has been underfinanced and resources are misallocated across diseases. The ten diseases that cause 76 percent of DLYs lost in Ethiopia consume total spending of only 45 percent of recurrent expenditures. The Government health care system has been highly centralized and reliant on vertical programs.

THE PROGRAM: OBJECTIVES AND STRATEGY

In response to these issues the Council of Ministers adopted a National Health Policy in September 1993. The Policy calls for decentralization of health services; development of preventive and promotional components of health care; assuring accessibility of health care for all segments of the population; mobilization of and maximal utilization of internal and external resources for development of the sector—including cost recovery on the basis of ability and promotion of private and non-government organizations in health care.

The National Health Policy was further developed and refined—in part with Bank assistance through a PHRD grant—and presented as a Health Sector Development Program (HSDP) at the Consultative Group Meeting of Donors in Addis Ababa in December 1996. This 20-year program seeks to develop a health system that provides comprehensive and integrated primary case services for all Ethiopians, primarily based at community health facilities. The focus is on communicable diseases, common nutritional disorders, environmental health and hygiene, reproductive health care, immunization, the

---

[1] Based on the Project Appraisal Document for a Health Sector Development Program, September 24, 1998, Report No. 18366-ET and interview with former Team Leader, Mr. David Berk.

TABLE 1

Health Status	Base (1997)	2002	2017
Life expectancy			
Overall 52	5	5-60	—
Males 49.7	56.2	—	
Females	52.4	59.2	—
Infant mortality rate (per 1,000 live births)	110-128	90-95	50
Maternal mortality rate (per 100,000 live births)	500-700	450-500	300
Health Services			
Expand primary health care coverage			
(% of population)	45	55-60	90
Immunization (DPT3) coverage	67	70-80	90
Contraceptive prevalence	8	15-20	40

treatment and control of basic infectious diseases, epidemic diseases, and sexually transmitted diseases.

The 20-year program (1997-2016) starts with a first phase of five years (July 1997-June 2002). An IDA-financed Health Sector Development Project provides the equivalent of US$100 million to support the first phase. Key indicators of progress in health status and services for the first phase and full 20-year implementation are set out in the table below:

The Government strategy to achieve these targets includes: decentralization of operational responsibilities through a four-tier system (primary health care units, district hospitals, regional hospitals, and specialized hospitals) based on defined minimum standards, greater public funding for health care, expansion of facilities into underserved areas, an emphasis on preventive care and community-based delivery of health services; and increased supply and logistics systems for essential drugs along with better quality assurance and better training for frontline and middle level health service providers. Accordingly, the first five-year phase of the HSDP includes the following components: (1) expansion of primary health care access through provision of facilities according to predefined physical norms, (2) improvements in the technical quality of service provision, (3) expanding the supply and productiv-

ity of health personnel, (4) improvements in the pharmaceutical sector, (5) information, education, and communication, (6) health sector management and management information systems, (7) monitoring and evaluation and applied research, and (8) improvements in the financial sustainability of the health sector through greater efficiency and mobilization of additional resources.

SWAP DESIGN

Bank Lending Instrument: Specific Investment Loan (SIL)

Rationale for the SWAP: A sector-wide approach was adopted to support the overall program. The climate of opinion in the Bank favored adoption of the sector-wide approach and the Government's initiative in preparing an overall sector policy suggested the need for a SWAP.

SWAP characteristics: The operation has at least five elements that have been identified with SWAPS, namely: (1) an overall policy framework, (2) an expenditure framework, (3) agreement by the main donors to the program, (4) the government had enough influence over the process to call it ownership, and (5) attempts at common implementation arrangements.

Preconditions: Ethiopia met several basic preconditions for starting the development of a sector-wide approach: It had achieved macroeconomic stability. Through previous investments it had demonstrated at least a minimum level of institutional capacity for program execution. Above all, it had demonstrated commitment to a sector-wide process through the definition of first its National Health Policy in 1993 and then the development of the HSDP by 1996.

Definition of the sector: A pragmatic decision was taken on the definition of the health sector for operational purposes, namely: whatever the Ministry of Health (MOH) dealt with. Thus, the sector is comprehensive rather than limited to certain subsectors, yet does not get into practical difficulties of cross-ministerial responsibilities. The "sector" is congruent with the existing management units for planning and budgeting.

Program leadership: By default leadership for the development of the sector program was vested on the government side in the Office of the Prime Minister (PMO). The Ministry of Health had lost substantial managerial capacity through a government-wide process of decentralization. Key staff either were moved to the regions or left the Ministry rather than be reassigned to regions. This left a capacity and leadership vacuum in the MOH. The Minister in charge of social sectors in the PMO was the former Minister of Health and was fully conversant with sectoral issues and requirements. On the side of the donors, in theory the donor group was the counterpart to the government. However, the Government asked the Bank to take the lead in the preparation of the program and lead the missions. Consultation between donors and Government was achieved through joint participation in the Sector Steering Committee, which included the Ministry of Finance and was chaired by the Minister in the PMO.

Program development: Program development included the following main stages: (1) formation of a Task Force to prepare a National Health Policy that was adopted in September 1993; (2) preparation of the HSDP, in part with Bank assistance, by December 1996; (3) presentation of the HSDP by the Government to the donor community at a workshop in March 1997 (together with the Education Sector Development Program), (4) Three multidonor missions (October 1997; February 1998; May 1998) which in effect were identification, preparation, and appraisal, but different terms were used. The Government produced a detailed Program Action Plan (PAP) for appraisal. Another key document, the Implementation Manual, was finalized by the Government after Board presentation. Donors were incorporated into the process relatively late in the game, by which time many basic parameters for the program had already been decided. The main substantive issue during the dialogue with donors was the composition of the capital and recurrent budgets. At the urging of the donors the Government saw that the original capital-heavy program could not be sustained. Changes were made to achieve a better balance between capital and recurrent expenditures.

Level of sector analysis: Development of the program benefited from several analyses. Two PHRD grants financed thirteen studies that provided input into the definition and refinement of the HSDP. However, the Government did not wait for the results of these studies before writing up its program. It is not clear whether the studies were ever drawn upon fully. In addition, the Bank undertook a Public Expenditure Review in 1997 and a Social Sector Review in 1998 that provided a basis, *inter alia*, for its economic analysis of the program.

Instruments for agreements: The Government prepared the documents (policies, plans and manuals) that set out objectives, means, and obligations. Donors agreed to provide support based on these documents. A specific Letter of Sector Policy was written and addressed to the Bank. Late in the process the idea was discussed of having a Memorandum of Understanding setting out responsibilities among the various participants. Government resisted the idea, saying they did not see the need given all the other documentation produced.

Institutional capacity: No special instruments were used to assess institutional capacity at the center or in the regions. The central MOH had been gutted by the departure or defection of key personnel during the process of decentralization. The MOH had no confidence in its ability to perform its new role of technical support to (without supervisory control over) regions. Donors established a condition for further processing of assistance that sector management be strengthened and improved. This was accomplished. Particular attention was devoted during appraisal to institutional capacity for procurement and financial management, including specialists in these fields in the missions.

Stakeholder consultation: Ethiopia has had an autocratic tradition. Authorities felt they "knew best" what should be done. Consistent with this, authorities were not much concerned with consultation with stakeholders and beneficiaries. There was a belated attempt to contact NGOs, but overall little was done. Donors did not challenge this approach. One consequence is a risk that the proposed approach to improved medical care at the local level may not be accepted, and expected increased utilization of services may not materialize.

Financing: IDA is providing US$100 million and other donors about $215 million for a five-year program that is expected to cost about $750 million. The Government, thus, will finance about 55% of total costs. The Bank is playing the role of the "lender of last resort," i.e., financing components left after other donors have chosen what to finance. This role is complicated because some donors—mainly for reasons of Ethiopia's war with Eritrea—have slowed or suspended their commitment of funds. It has also meant by default that the Bank will finance a high proportion of the civil works component. This was considered acceptable since the civil works is part of a well-defined overall expenditure framework directed at high-priority objectives. Also, civil works is not the only component that the Bank will finance. Schedule 1 of the Credit Agreement leaves 65% of the credit proceeds in the unallocated category to promote flexibility in allocations. This allows funds to be shifted quickly from activities that are not doing well to others that are, or to activities of greatest need at the time.

Procurement: The Credit Agreement required national competitive bidding according to national procedures for most procurement, with thresholds set relatively high. Attempts have been made to develop standard bidding documents and processes in a way that would be acceptable for use by other donors. It is expected that some of the donors will agree on common thresholds for procurement methods and reporting formats at the post-review level, thus reducing MOH's administrative burden. Donors may also agree on the use of standard documents and procedures for advertising, evaluating, and awarding contracts.

Disbursements: Funds are not pooled under the Program. HSDP financial management uses the existing channels: The Ministry of Finance passes funds from both central government and donors (kept separately) to the central MOH and to regional offices of the MOF, where regional offices of the MOH will obtain their share of total regional funds. A single set of accounts in agreed format show all sources and uses of funds for HSDP at each level. Thus, IDA will make disbursements against eligible expenditures based on statements of expenditure (SOEs) or full documentation for payments above SOE thresholds. IDA will advance funds into a central government Special Account for IDA's share of program expenditures. Project accounts have also been opened in each of the regions to cover IDA's share of the annual work program and budget.

Risks and dangers as a SWAP: The magnitude of the sector program means that it is more vulnerable to macro shocks than would be a smaller project (for which some funds could normally be found to finance its continuation.) If this happens, it would mean doing less, i.e., scaling down tertiary health facility targets, or slowing down capital expenditures so as to reduce associated recurrent expenditures. Another risk is that donors may not provide resources as intended. This risk appears to have been realized because several donors have slowed contributions in response to the war. Another issue concerns implementation capacity. Since the Ministry of Health has to do or supervise all procurement, rather than multiple PIUs as would be the case under separate donor projects, its implementation capacity is strained. Another complication of the SWAP approach is getting financial flows the way everyone wants them.

Conditionality: Conditions of effectiveness include preparation of the Project Implementation Manual, and adoption of an acceptable plan to strengthen financial management. It took an exceptionally long time to declare the credit, largely because of the difficulty in reaching an acceptable financial management plan. Conditions of disbursement on subprograms include (1) (a) prior IDA approval of the subprogram, and (b) preparation of an operational plan for the subprogram (including reforms, activities, financing required, sources of financing, and a procurement plan), and (2) satisfactory evidence that (a) the budget for the subprogram is consistent with overall Program objectives, and (b) previous expenditures were made in compliance with Program objectives. In effect, implementation of the annually agreed program is a condition for commitments from year to year. The financing levels are highly flexible. If the Government reduces its level of financing of the Program (as appears to be now emerging), IDA reduces its financing. Poor results from one year can lead to reduced new financing for the next year. No other special remedies are incorporated into the legal agreement.

SWAP IMPLEMENTATION

Organizational arrangements: The HSDP is implemented by the central Ministry of Health and Regional Bureaus of Health (about 90% of the expenditures are below the central level). Coordination is provided by a Central Joint Steering Committee (CJSC) and Regional Joint Steering Committees. The CJSC is chaired by the Senior Minister for Social and Administrative Affairs in the PMO. Other members include the Ministers of Finance, Economic Development and Cooperation, Health, Education and three donor representatives (currently the Bank, UNDP, and USAID.) The Planning and Projects Department of the MOH serves as secretariat to the CJSC.

Modus operandi and instruments used: Targets exist for the various subprograms, but it is not known in advance what specific components will be financed, where, and when. These specific funding decisions are to be made during the course of implementation based on annual programs and budgets, overall and by region. Key to this is the joint Government donor annual review. The annual review examines actual achievements and performance under the program of the previous year and decides on the budget and targets for the next year. Annual reviews allow the work program to be adjusted according to past performance and changing circumstances. In turn, a key requirement for the annual review is development of the management information system of the MOH. Semiannual Implementation Progress Reports are being submitted by implementing agencies covering: (1) expenditure data from the previous six months; (2) data on physical targets achieved (and actual achievements as a percentage of targets); (3) procurement status report and plan for the next two years; (4) issues and problems; (5) action plan to resolve the problems. Reports by regions and the center are then integrated into a consolidated report for consideration by the Central Steering Committee (CSC). The Annual Review Package, in addition, includes information on monitorable indicators, review of priorities and strategies, reports on special studies and updated work programs and proposed budgets. Efforts have also been made to harmonize donor procedures. Donors have agreed to work together to harmonize the financial accounting and management systems. The long term goal is to have all donors use Government channels for the flow of program funds and reporting.

Implementation experience: The Program has been under implementation since 1997, before the IDA Credit of $100 million was approved. One annual review has been held since IDA Credit approval. The initial annual review turned out to be less than satisfactory. The implementing agencies produced generally weak progress reports. After much discussion about indicators and reporting systems, the management information system is not yet installed even after two years of Program implementation. Another problem detected is the poor organization and procedures to follow up on new government commitments. Another problem has been the reluctance of some donors to meet their commitments—because of the war, particularly those donors who previously had been for more general budget support. There have been few disagreements among donors and government on policy matters—mainly because the worldwide consensus that exists in the health sector on strategic priorities and means of intervention.

gram was able to learn from the experiences of the education program, which was developed on a schedule about six months ahead of health. The health program used the same cycle of mission, for example. As a result, the health program started work on implementation aspects earlier than education. The health program also addressed the issue of management capacity in the MOH early, during the preparation process. Finally, in general, the process of donor coordination and involvement through the Steering Committee and annual reviews has proved to be workable.

OUTCOMES SO FAR

Main achievements: (1) Rebalancing sector expenditures, i.e., reducing the excessive capital expenditures to achieve a more proper balance with recurrent expenditures and increase the likelihood of financial sustainability. (2) The Government now understands more fully what goes into a sector program. In particular, the regions have undergone an extensive learning process in terms of preparing regional plans. (3) The MOH has a stronger setup for implementation. (4) The Government has learned how to deal with donors and their foibles. The health pro-

LESSONS

The following lessons should be noted:

(1) Donors should become involved earlier in the process of program development, before Government has made up its mind on key aspects.
(2) Proper stakeholder consultations should take place, and stakeholders should have a greater role in the steering groups.
(3) Get donors to commit to move together with financing.

TABLE 2
756 - ETHIOPIA , HEALTH SECTOR
Project Status Report Date: 6/24/99

Region:	AFR	Country: ETHIOPIA			Sector:	HB	Lending Instr:	SIL
Prg Obj Cat:	PA	EA Cat: B	PTI?	Y	NGO?	N	Resettlement?	N

LOAN INFORMATION

Agree Type	L/C/G No.	Orig Amt	Rev'd Amt	Currency Indicator	Prod Line	Signing Date	Effective Date	Suppl Prj ID
IDA	31400	75.10 (SDR)			PE	10/30/98	3/11/99	

Total Original Amount (SDR): 75.10   Total Revised Amount (SDR): 0.00

COFINANCING INFORMATION

Agency	Board Amount ($M)	Current Amount ($M)
Total	0.00	0.00

Guarantee Type: Guarantee Amount ($M):

This form is part of: **Portfolio status update**

Read together with:

( ) Aide-memoire   Mission End Date: This Form PSR Date: 6/24/99
( ) BTO memo of: Months since last mission: Last Form PSR Date: 1/22/99
( ) Follow-up letter of: Next mission planned:

SUPERVISION EFFORT

	Total Staff-Weeks	Total $000	Field Staff-weeks	Field $000	As of 6/24/99
Current FY - Planned	21.80	85.92			
Current FY - Actual	29.85	93.52	0.00	0.00	
Board through preceding FY	0.00	0.00	0.00	0.00	
Total Actual	29.85	93.52	0.00	0.00	

UPI No.	Mission Member	Division	No. of Fld Days	Role or Specialization	PrevMiss

Ghana Health Case Study[1]
Health Sector Support Program

ACRONYMS

BMC   Budget and Management Center (functionally and administratively accountable units)

GHS   Ghanaian Health Service

HSSP   Health Sector Support Program

MOH   Ministry of Health

MOU   Memorandum of Understanding

MTHS   Medium-Term Health Strategy toward Vision 2020 (The Policy Framework)

POW   Five-Year Program of Work, 1997-2001 (The Operational Framework)

SAR   Staff Appraisal Report

BACKGROUND

Health and population outcomes and service provision indicators are slightly better in Ghana than the average for Sub-Saharan Africa with mortality trends improving at a faster pace. Since independence in the early 1960s life expectancy has increased from 45 to 55 years. Ghana has one of the more advanced health systems in Africa, including a relatively strong district health management system. Yet the health status of Ghanaians is still poor: the infant mortality rate is about 66 per 1000, the total fertility rate is 5.5, about 8 percent of children under 5 years suffer from severe malnutrition, and large disparities exist between regions, particularly in the north. According to the 1998 Ghana Demographic and Health survey, infant mortality is 56 per 1000 (with neonatal and post-neonatal deaths respectively at 29 and 27 per 1000). Under-five mortality is 107 per 1000 births, having significantly decreased (30% in the last 15 years). Fertility has declined dramatically over the last decade from over 6 births per woman in the mid-1980s to 4.5 births per woman during the last five years. At current fertility rates, women in rural areas will have nearly twice as many children (5.4) as women in urban areas (3.0). About 40 percent of the population still does not have access to health facilities and 50% do not have access to safe water. Utilization of curative services is quite low, with only 0.39 annual visits per capita in public facilities. Quality is constrained by shortages of supplies, absence of services, questionable staff behavior and absence of quality assurance programs and beneficiary feedback. In the mid-1990s Government expenditures on health declined, particularly for non-wage recurrent expenditures. Rather than targeting the poor, Government resources have been disproportionately spent on less cost-effective tertiary levels of curative care. (President's Report: 2.)

---

[1] Based on interviews with Mr. Francois Decaillet, detailed comments by David Peters and the documents cited at the end of the case study.

A health reform program was articulated in a Medium-Term Health Strategy: toward Vision 2020 (MTHS). The four sector policy guidelines for resource allocation are to (a) make more resources available for attainment of universal access to primary health services and shift the emphasis increasingly to the primary level; (b) increase the share of non-wage items in the total recurrent budget; (c) achieve a better balance between development and recurrent budgets; and (d) realign existing inequalities in regional allocations.

The Bank had two previous credits dealing solely or in part with health. About 15 donors and technical agencies had been active in providing assistance to the health sector, contributing just under 30% of public expenditures on health. One of the major problems prior to the MTHS was the lack of an overall framework for integrating the many donor-assisted projects. Investment decisions were made in isolation, there were many vertical programs and parallel management systems, and a lack of congruence of project aims. These tended to fragment rather than build capacity. Coordination of activities of donors and technical agencies, as well as multiple reporting requirements, was becoming increasingly unmanageable and disruptive to Government.

SWAP DESIGN

Lending instrument: The project is classified as a Sector Investment Loan (SIL) and was used informally as a test case for an Adaptable Program Loan (APL). The project is clearly a Sector Investment Program because it meets the following criteria: (1) sector-wide in scope; (2) based on an overall policy and expenditure framework; (3) Government leadership and ownership of the program; (4) donors financed a share of the investment program and agreed to harmonize procedures; (5) use of government institutions and procedures for implementation of the program; and (6) minimal use of long- term external technical assistance.

Rationale for the SWAP: According to the SAR, one of the reasons for selection of the sector pro-

gram versus a project approach is to improve sustainability (p. 21). Under the sector approach all financial requirements and funding sources are considered in one envelope. The capital investment program is scrutinized carefully, including implications on recurrent expenditures. Agreement on levels of financing and monitoring actual performance against those targets help to ensure that the program will be financially sustainable. Institutional sustainability will be enhanced by focusing on improved management practices and support to regular institutions and processes rather than separate project structures and donor-based processes. In addition, the comprehensive sector approach, founded on a basic package of services designed to balance cost-effectiveness and equity, was seen as a means to achieve greater impact in solving chronic problems in the sector. The Bank wanted to support the Ghanaian-led initiative on health reforms. It provided a forum to consider openly a full range of public policy and allocation issues, and adopt common goals and strategies. In contrast, traditional projects diverted implementation capacity and duplicated efforts, lowering the chances for sustainability and coordinating financing with sector priorities (SAR, p. 8).

Context: The HSSP benefited from a history that was conducive for a sector-wide approach. First, the Government had achieved substantial macroeconomic stability in the 1980s through its economic recovery program. Despite setbacks in the early 1990s, growth was strong in the mid 1990s, including a 5.2 percent increase in GDP in 1996 and a reduction in inflation from 71 percent at the end of 1995 to 29 percent by June 1997. Second, the Government had demonstrated considerable institutional capacity through its earlier reforms in the health sector, including the establishment of district health services, development of financial management systems, and successful implementation of numerous externally financed assistance programs. In short, an administrative and institutional basis existed on which to build. Third, the Government had led the process of defining a long-term policy and strategy for health sector reform and, by definition, claimed strong ownership for them.² Despite the progress it had achieved, problems in health care were still massive, suggesting the need for a new approach with greater impact.

Definition of the sector: The definition of the sector for the health program is comprehensive. It covers all activities in the health sector. This ranges from individual and household health decisions to formal service delivery, advocacy, institutional arrangements, and policy addressing public and private providers and other stakeholders and beneficiaries of the health sector. The financing of the program cover all Government and donor-assisted activities, both recurrent and developmental, so that all input can be directed toward common objectives (SAR, p. 9). In terms of other sector plans, such as nutrition and population control, the Plan of Work (POW) specifies what operational responsibilities would be included. For example, the health services elements of nutrition strategies (e.g., prevention and control of micronutrient deficiency) are included. Food security initiatives are not part of the health sector POW. Communications, essential obstetric services and management of sexually transmitted diseases are part of the health interventions included in the POW (SAR, p. 10). Essentially the POW covers all activities controlled by the Ministry of Health and the Ghanaian Health Service. (In addition, several ministries were involved in approval, consultation, and division of labor. Finance, Planning, Control and Accountant General, Auditor General, and Head of Civil Service were needed for "approval" on different aspects of the program. Consultation was needed from many Ministries (e.g., education, etc.), and a division of labor was needed with Ministries of Local Government and Environment).

Program leadership: The Government itself decided to adopt a sector-wide approach to overcome fragmentation of projects, which results in a heavier burden on the Government. Donor agencies assisted in the development of the strategies and programs but the Government was very much in the driver's seat for the entire process. The leadership tended to be exercised by a relatively small number of senior officials in the central MOH.³ Leadership emanated from the Minister of Health who initiated the process, but was soon taken over by a group including the Director General, the Director of Policy, Planning, Monitoring and Evaluation, and a few key Directors (External Aid, Human Resources, Health Research Unit). However, the emphasis was on giving more authority and responsibility to Regional Directors and District Medical Officers, creating local changes and power bases.

Donor coordination: A forum for donors and some NGOs was in existence for decades in Ghana, but had not succeeded in overcoming the perceived constraints on coordination. Donors stuck to their systems and procedures and insisted on being identified with particular projects. From the Government perspective separate donor projects afforded individuals the opportunity to command and control selected programs and benefits, e.g., study tours abroad. However, small groups of donors in the MOH responded to the ever more pressing need for coordination brought on by the multiple demands imposed by projects and the need for a more coherent sector plan to achieve vital development objectives (Annan: 5). At present monthly meetings are held for the Government-donor coalition. Better coordination was achieved by a number of steps: changing the chairmanship of the coordination group over

---

² This occurred more during the course of preparation than as a precondition to undertaking the approach. Project staff stated that one should avoid too much reference to preconditions. When starting dialogue about SWAPs one is setting out development objectives instead of prerequisites.

³ One reviewer noted, a close relationship existed between a small group of health sector donors and a core of senior MOH personnel. From 1996 onwards technical assistance was provided to introduce the sector-wide program. "The principal effects of donor funding on local ownership of strategies were the acquiescence to specific donor preferences" (Annan, p. ii).

to Government; conducting joint missions, preparing joint TOR, dividing up the work, and frequent formal and informal consultations. In addition, informal consultations were frank, open exchanges, which have persisted to this day. The main factor was the openness of the Ghanaians to discussing any issue.

Program development: The MTHS was developed after a National Consultative Meeting on Health Development in late 1993. This was followed by 14 working groups to further develop feasible strategies. A Steering Committee then consolidated the wide variety of inputs into the MTHS. "Donors and technical agencies, led by the World Bank, agreed in principle that supporting a common Sector Investment Program based on the Government's health sector strategy was the way of the future. ... To this end, the health donors agreed to support the MOH in evolving a five-year Program of Work from the Strategy. Paradoxically, to reach this turning point where partners were 'on board', it had taken nearly three years of fragmented project type arrangements to support the sector-wide approach" (Annan: 8). After the painful process of getting out the MTHS, the POW was basically formed by following the discipline of the new budgeting and planning cycle. A new budget and plan were required, so that efforts were first made to get each BMC to produce its plan and budget, and then to pull them together at the national level. It is difficult in retrospect to identify any clear-cut stages for IDA in getting to negotiations and Board approval. There were consultations and meetings, and considerable back and forth on the agreements reached. These included numerous meetings between Legal, Disbursement, Bank Procurement advisors, and the AFPH4 team. At one point the project staff met with some concerned Executive Directors over the procurement issues. The project was also taken to the Regional Operations Committee, and the main Operations Committee, to formally review the project before negotiations and the Board. The main disagreements on policy during program design concerned the capital budget, which needed to be reduced to focus less on hos-

pital care and be balanced better with recurrent financing. In terms of modalities the most difficult areas for agreement were on financial management and procurement procedures, especially the pooling of donor funds.

Level of sector analysis: There was considerable sector analysis already done—on health status, on health determinants, on NGOs, beneficiary assessments, etc. Bank staff added a procurement assessment, an assessment of financial management (and specific review of each BMC for clearance), an institutional assessment, and a public health assessment.

Instruments for agreements: The Government's plans and programs provided the basic instruments for agreements, particularly the POW and annual work programs. Late in the design stage, after approval of the IDA Credit, a Memorandum of Understanding was signed by other donors along with a Code of Practice. These documents were used to specify the roles and responsibilities of the Government and donors during implementation. Other key instruments used included joint aide memoires (with other donors and government), joint mission TORs, and agreement on a single set of monitoring reports.

Institutional capacity: Institutional assessment was done in 1994, and supplemented by other assessments of specific parts of the institution and its beneficiaries as was needed.

Stakeholder consultation: According to the President's Report considerable consultations took place in the design and initial implementation of the HSSP. Both the Consultative Meeting and the working groups had broad representation of stakeholders in public and private sectors in Ghana. Outside the MOH, active partnership is being sought with missions, other NGOs and private practitioners, suppliers of goods and services, universities, and research institutions. There have also been increasing efforts to involve health consumers in health reform discussions. Studies on user satisfaction indicate a movement within MOH to assess client expectations. Efforts are being made to make the reform as broad-based and populist as possible (pp. 8, 10). Another review, however, states that non-health and non-state actors were poorly represented in the planning and implementation of the sector-wide program, and there was little "grassroots" input. "As a result of the limited stakeholder participation, the priorities and local needs identified, which require a broad consensus, lack full legitimacy" (Annan: 9). "Though leadership was provided, it was not apparent that the sector-wide process through its top-down approach had increased professional ownership beyond a small group" (Annan: 27). "The MOH recognized the need to build consensus around its strategy, but this proved elusive largely due to the donor-induced haste to develop a more fundable Program of Work" (Annan: ii).

THE PROGRAM

Objectives and content: The HSSP seeks to implement the MTHS, as defined more specifically in the five-year Program of Work (POW). The ultimate aim is to improve the health status of Ghanaians. The two main goals of the reform program are to: (a) provide universal access to a basic package of health services and improve the quality and efficiency of health services; and (b) foster linkages with other sectors to reduce population growth rates, reduce the level of malnutrition, etc. Program impact targets are as follows:

The POW presents seven strategies with content as follows: (1) improving the access, quality, and efficiency of primary health services by establishing standards of practice for a priority package of services, retraining health workers, rehabilitating clinics, health centers and district hospitals, providing essential drugs, equipment and supplies according to standardized lists, and strengthening management and administrative systems in the decentralized system; (2) strengthening and reorienting secondary and tertiary service delivery to support primary care; (3) training adequate numbers of new health teams, including in-service training, expanded and restructured pre-service training, rehabilitation of schools, provision of supplies and teaching materials, revision of curricula and retraining tutors; (4) improving the capacity of the MOH for policy development and analysis, resource allocation and performance monitoring and regulation of service delivery; (5) strengthening national support systems for personnel management, supplies management, and financial management and health information; (6) promoting private sector involvement in health service delivery, including development of contractual arrangements, regulatory, and licensing mechanisms; and (7) strengthening intersectoral collaboration in terms of advocacy for nutritional and population programs.

Organization for implementation: The long-term vision is to use common implementation arrangements for the public sector, regardless of the source of the funding. This entails developing and strengthening existing systems rather than building

TABLE 1

Indicator	Baseline	Target 2001
Life expectancy (years)	58	60
Infant mortality (deaths per 1,000 live births)	66	50
Under-five mortality (per 1,000 live births)	132	100
Maternal mortality (per 100,000 live births	214	100
Annual population growth (percent)		2.75
Total fertility rate (births)	5.5	5.0
Children with severe malnutrition (percent)	12	8

Source: Staff Appraisal Report, p. 9.

separate systems for each project. The program, therefore, is being implemented through the regular channels of the Government. No new project implementation units have been established. The MOH is responsible for policy, monitoring, coordination of donors, and public financing for health services. As a transition toward single Government systems over time, in the medium term the program is being managed by tightly coordinated parallel and common implementation arrangements for those with existing projects. The Ghana Health Service and two Teaching Hospital Boards are managing the delivery of public health services in a decentralized context. They prepare and implement health budgets and monitor health performance. Responsibility and authority for service delivery are delegated to various BMCs, including 110 district health management teams that are responsible for organizing and providing local health services. Ten regional health teams play an intermediary role between the district teams and the central GHS (SAR: p. 22).

Modus operandi: Common methods have been developed for financial management, auditing, procurement, management of logistics and technical assistance, monitoring, and reporting. Common implementation arrangements have been outlined in a Memorandum of Understanding (MOU, 30 April 1999) between the Government and donors.[4] The MOU contains many of the provisions of the Development Credit Agreement with the Bank, including overall targets for Government financing of the health sector, exclusion of activities outside the agreed POW, appraisal of new capital projects, common procurement procedures, common disbursement procedures, minimum "readiness criteria" for disbursement of funds to BMCs, appointment of an acceptable independent auditor, and the annual schedule of work. In addition, a "Code of Practice" is attached to the MOU that stresses sharing of information; increasing responsibility for technical assistance by the MOH; channeling all earmarked, project-specific funds through the Financial Controller rather than directly to program managers; prohibition of independent monitoring visits by cooperating partners; and MOH responsibility for planning annual reviews.

All planning and budgeting are now being done on the same schedule and not separately for each donor-funded activity. Government and donors jointly review the detailed action and financing plans at a national level on an annual basis. Two annual meetings are held by the MOH with donors and technical agencies. The first, in about April is called the "Health Summit" and concerns an annual assessment of performance and audit of the previous year. An extensive joint review is conducted by the Government and representatives of donor agencies prior to the Health Summit. The outcome of the Summit is a set of priorities and budget ceilings for the next year. The second meeting, in September, is limited to agencies providing flexible Program Financing, and it concerns financing commitments prior to the Ministry's submission of its budget to the Ministry of Finance. (See Timetable of Major Health Sector Planning and Monitoring Events, President's Report, Schedule B, Table 1). In addition, a monthly Government-Health Partners meeting keeps participants updated about current issues and enables them to discuss operational matters. Districts and regions report quarterly on problems and accomplishments. Before the end of 2001 a major evaluation of progress of the POW is planned, including an explicit measurement of health impact. Bank supervision focuses on assisting the MOH and GHS with problem solving, particularly on systemic issues and policy concerns. This means the Bank must keep up to date about how health services are operating at different levels, how beneficiaries are affected, and what other partners are doing. The Bank sends teams to both semiannual meetings and conducts assessments and spot checks on the measurement of performance indicators before the April meeting. It focuses particu-

---

[4] The Bank is not a signatory to the MOU since most of its provisions are included in the Development Credit Agreement.

larly on issues related to macroeconomic linkages, health financing and procurement, areas in which it took a leading role in the preparation and appraisal process. Other missions can be called by the Government and donors to deal with specific issues. The Bank also maintains a local resident mission presence to keep abreast of sector developments and to continue the dialogue.

Procurement: The exact mix of civil works, good and services to be financed is based on the annual plans of the POW. At the time of Board approval, the Government and MOH were currently putting into place procurement procedures acceptable to IDA and other donors, in particular responding to the recommendations of a Joint MOH-Donors Procurement Mission in October 1996. The memorandum of understanding (MOU) outlines the common procurement procedures to be followed under the Health Account. Some donors would continue following their own procurement procedures, but these practices would be phased out over time (SAR, pp. 24-5). To focus efforts on improving sustainable procurement systems within Ghana to cover multiple sources of funds, an independent third-party review would be the major source of procurement review, rather than a review by the Bank. An *a posteriori* third-party review would become the main method of review. However, IDA prior reviews would be applied to all international competitive bidding (ICB) packages in excess of US$2 million, goods over $300,000 and consultant contracts over $100,000 if the financing involves IDA funds in whole or in part (SAR, p. 27). A procurement plan indicates the source of financing. The Health Account, which includes IDA funds and others, is a source for some of the procurement contracts. It is not earmarked by the donors putting the money into the Health Account. Nor can the individual donors be identified for contracts paid from the Health Account, except as a proportion of the funds.

Financing: The first five years of the sector program is estimated to cost about US$825 million, of which about US$200 million (24%) would be financed by external donors, 70% by the Government, and the balance from cost recovery. Fifteen donors

and the Bank are supporting the Program. All financing would occur within the boundaries of the POW; the Government has agreed not to accept any financing outside this context. An IDA Credit for US$35 million provides a base amount of US$7 million per year. An interesting feature of the Credit is the possibility to vary annual disbursements in relation to performance. Conditions for baseline funding include (a) the Government meets its fiscal commitments to financing the POW, and (b) audits of the POW demonstrate adequate fiscal probity (SAR, p. 18). If these conditions are not met, the Bank would decrease IDA amounts below the baseline. Flexibility also exists to increase the amounts disbursed based on three additional conditions: (a) capacity to implement the POW as measured by ability to spend according to POW plans; (b) an increasing gap between the budget and available grant funds in which case IDA funds could be used to fill the gap; and (c) strong showing on the agreed set of sector performance indicators. In the future it is expected that financing will be explicitly linked to performance on agreed sector indicators (SAR, p. 18). Consistent with this flexibility, Schedule 1 of the Credit Agreement leaves US$30 million of $35 million (86%) unallocated. Funds are available for all non-wage categories of expenditure except taxes and land acquisition. The SAR describes the prospect of "gap filling" in external funds as IDA playing the role of donor of last resort. In view of the long-term nature of building capacity in the health sector, the continuing need for external financing, and the long time required to improve the health status of a population, IDA could make a long-term commitment in the form of a series of Credits. Upon disbursement of 75% of the existing Credit, the Bank would seek follow-up Credits based on the evaluation of performance under the POW (SAR, pp. 17, 33).

Flow of funds and disbursements: A unique feature of the IDA Credit is the use of a common account and pooling of resources. The SAR states that the MOH has gone a long way to establish financial management systems that will ensure appropriate use and accounting of funds (p. 22). The majority of donor funds, including the IDA Credit, will be managed on lines of existing government procedures. Some earmarked project funds will continue over the medium term, but the preferred donor financing system is an untied contribution into a common Health Account. Once IDA and other donor funds reach the Health Account, there is no further identification of the funds by donor origins, thus the funds are genuinely pooled. (SAR, p. 23). IDA is putting all its resources into the pool. Three other donors[5] are putting part of their contributions into the pool. The rest of the resources and those of other donors are earmarked funds, but are not provided in the traditional manner, as they are planned according to the annual planning and budgeting cycle, and are channeled through the Financial Controller in an accountable manner, rather than directly to program managers in isolation of other funding.[6] The Health Account funds are put into a bank account under the direct control of MOH and the Controller and Accountant General. These funds are then distributed to all eligible BMCs that meet minimum "Readiness Criteria", including: (1) submission of annual budget accompanied by quantified targets and objectives; (2) satisfactory procedures and collecting and accounting for independently generated funds; (3) adequate procedures for authorization of payments; (4) adequate and timely maintenance of accounts; and (5) adequate staff and procedures to prepare monthly reports on revenues and expenditures (SAR, p. 24).

One of the issues in program development was whether to reimburse against receipts or disburse against outcomes. The latter is the intention, but the former is the transitional arrangement. IDA reimburses expenditures already incurred out of government funds for the health sector based on the submission of financial management reports under the POW, including supporting documentation for the usual IDA withdrawal applications. Disbursements are made approximately every quarter. (A condition of disbursement includes the submission of the annual MOH budget submitted to parliament. In addition, meeting the "Readiness Criteria" is a precondition for the disbursement of Health Accounts funds by the MOH to a BMC. In the view of Bank staff the "disbursement issue" exists only because of Bank requirements. MOH regularly produces and certifies the required financial statements. Other donors are disbursing on the basis of these statements only.

Auditing of funds: Under current procedures the MOH is audited annually by the Auditor General and this would continue under the project. In addition, an acceptable private firm is hired under subcontract with the Auditor General to provide verification that all payments out of the Health Account (not just donor funds) have been used in accordance with the POW. Major BMCs are to be audited each year and others at least every three years depending on size. An acceptable audit report each year, by July 1, is a condition for maintenance of Bank funds at the base level for the following year. Independent audits have been conducted on finances, financial management, and procurement. It is worth noting that these audits cover all HSSP funds and procurement, not only donor contributions.

Risks: The SAR identifies several risks associated with financing the HSSP. First, decentralization of budgeting and financial management risks mismanagement of donor (and Government) funds, particularly in view of the limited experience of BMCs in managing funds. This risk is minimized by limiting allocations to a set of BMCs that are certified to manage funds based on their capacity and auditing them regularly. Second, the Government may not

---

[5] Dutch assistance, DANIDA and DFID.

[6] However, the Code of Conduct states that these earmarked funds should be channeled through the Financial Controller rather than directly to program managers so as to enable the MOH to track total donor contributions and assist with annual planning and budgeting.

maintain its financing commitments to the POW, or may introduce questionable capital expenditures. This risk is managed by the provision to respond in the worst case (short of suspension or cancellation) by decreasing the amount to be allocated that year. Third, there is a risk that common implementation procedures with donors may not work. To deal with this risk a regular Government-donor forum has been established to monitor progress, and a MOU clarifies responsibilities. An informal Code of Conduct has also been drafted for guidance in other areas of interaction.

Annan identified some local perceptions of other risks in SWAPs: (a) "failure of policy dialogue could lead to a form of 'gridlock' for the sector; (b) donor influence could increase as a result of joint reviews and closer monitoring of policy outcomes; (c) flexibility and responsiveness could be limited due to the 'blueprint' nature of the program which, in essence, is not an evolving strategic plan; and (d) donors not involved are likely to perpetuate the problems of fungibility of aid and overburden government management capacity" (p. iv).

Conditions: The Government agreed during negotiations to take all actions to increase the levels of its expenditures on the health sector as agreed within the POW, including not less than 6.9% of Government recurrent expenditures in FY1997, 8.6% in FY1998, 9.5 percent in FY1999, 10.0 percent in FY2000, and 11.0 percent in FY2001. It also agreed to subject all proposed capital projects to appraisal according to agreed criteria; to submit an annual implementation plan and budget prior to the annual meeting with donors in September and review progress on the previous year's health plan; submit reports and financial statements covering achievement of indicators and use of POW funds before April each year for the joint Government-donor review, and lead a major evaluation of the POW before the end of the fifth year (SAR, pp. 32-33).

SWAP IMPLEMENTATION

Implementation experience: As indicated in the Bank supervision report[7] following the second annual review the Government has made good progress in implementing the POW. The Government has increased the percentage of the total recurrent budget spent on health from 7% in 1996 to 8.4% in 1997 and 8.6% in 1998—in accordance with POW targets. This was accompanied by a shift toward more decentralized funding and increase in internally generated funds. The public health services have shown improvements in terms of vaccinations and family planning services and a recent increase in outpatient services. Noticeable progress has been achieved in financial management and most of the 1998 objectives for procurement services have been achieved. The extensive review of performance in 1998 reported that "significant steps continue to be made to shape the reform process in policy and strategic terms and in capacity building, and in service delivery most of all." However, in other respects 1998 was a difficult year. The Minister of Health, the Director of the Medical Service, and other persons responsible for the reforms changed during the year. In addition, a review of the capital budget led to protracted disagreements over two hospital development programs. In the end an agreement was reached on the hospital rehabilitation projects (one being kept at the original allocation of $12 million and the other being re-assessed.) However, the disagreement and some administrative delays prevented some donors from disbursing into the health account. Donor contributions to earmarked programs were actually less in 1998 than in 1997. Despite these difficulties, the program has been implemented largely on schedule. Based on overall positive results, the Bank team recommended consideration for increasing the IDA allocation for FY2000 from the baseline amount of $7 million to $9 million, pending issuance of the final procurement and financial

---

[7] Francois Decaillet, Back-to-office report, June 1, 1999.

audits for 1998. The annual review was informed by an excellent comprehensive report prepared jointly by the Government and outside experts. People from the opposition party participated in the Health Summit in 1999. Other points include the following:

(1) Both annual reviews have commented upon the difficulties of getting good information on the indicators, although data for 1998 were much better than 1997. There was some dissatisfaction expressed about the indicators used and a need for a "thorough revision of these indicators to improve the performance contract system" (Supervision report, p. 2).

(2) It has taken longer than expected to get an acceptable Government procurement plan and reach agreement with the Auditor General about an independent auditor. The AG did not want outside interference. Eventually agreement was reached on a one-year contract with a private firm rather than a three-year contract as envisaged in the documents.

(3) An issue has also arisen in terms of inconsistency between the intention of using (improved) government procedures for procurement so as to build capacity, and the Development Credit Agreement that calls for Bank control of all procedures. The issue pertained to initial implementation, but has reportedly been resolved since receipt of the procurement audit report. It is now clear that the Bank's role is not to control, but help MOH to strengthen its own procurement and control capacities.

(4) A compromise was reached that reimbursements will be made against receipts and normal withdrawal applications; and that procurement will be controlled by the Bank. At the end of the year, and based on audits of both finances and procurement the procedures will be reconsidered. The Country Director can authorize changes.

(5) The review of other donor-assisted projects that fall outside the agreed program was an awkward and difficult process for donors, who are not accustomed to influencing the exclusion of projects supported by other donors.

(6) Another event during implementation that has the potential to slow reforms has been a strike by young doctors. Resolving the strike became a priority for the Government and the donor consortium also had to be concerned with the issue. Normally, with a project approach, the donors would not consider such events if they did not impinge on the specific projects being financed.

The coalition survived the change of the ministerial team, a conflict over the capital development program (Tamale and Koforidua hospital), the very turbulent situation created by unrest in the sector (strikes for better condition and against the militarization of hospitals in Accra), and the presentation of the procurement audit, which revealed some anomalies. An open, pragmatic, and cautious approach to dialogue is making this coalition strong.

OUTCOMES SO FAR

Main achievements:

(1) As noted in the Appraisal Report, a major benefit of the sector approach is already seen in improvements in the processes and results of policy dialogue and health sector planning. For the first time health policies are being explicitly linked to resource allocation in a comprehensive manner, covering all Government and donor financing. The sector approach has brought a more rational policy discussion and improved transparency and accountability. (SAR, p. 30).

(2) During the development of the sector-wide program the Government defined for the first time its overall capital program for the

health sector. After an initial agreement with donors on a capital program of US$230 million with priority given to primary health care, other parallel capital investments emerged that were outside the agreed program. These included the construction of regional hospitals financed by commercial loans and supplier credits. The total capital investment ballooned to $509 million and distorted the balance among levels and types of health care, and between planned recurrent and capital expenditures. This became a significant part of the macroeconomic dialogue between the Bank, the IMF, and Government, which eventually led to revisions of the capital program. A capital program of US$298 million was finally agreed on between the Government and donors (SAR, p. 15). In addition, new procedures for appraisal and procurement of capital programs were agreed on to prevent such occurrences in the future. This potential distortion in overall capital expenditures would not have been picked up without a sector-wide approach (SAR, p. 31).

Ghana is in the early stages of implementing many of its reforms, so it is still early to judge their impact. However, there are already indications of progress in the 20 annual performance indicators. (See Table.) Independent reviews of sector performance have also found the following progress and problems:

❖ *Transparency:* The level of transparency has greatly increased as a result of the annual review process. In addition, independent financial and management audits of the MOH were conducted in 1997 and 1998, and will continue to be conducted annually.

❖ *Reproductive health:* The number of family planning "couple years of protection" has increased. Knowledge and support for reproductive health are high, and Ghana has had *National Reproductive Health Service*

Policy and Standards since 1996. However, they remain largely unimplemented.

❖ *Quality of care:* Quality assurance teams are functional in five of the nine regional hospitals and partially functional in one other. Quarterly monitoring of quality assurance indicators has been carried out in several regions.

Main problems (or lack of achievements):
Specific issues identified during the 1998 annual performance review include:

❖ *MOH institutional capacity:* (1) There is a backlog of policies, strategies, plans, and protocols that have not been implemented. (2) The Management Information System has not been able to deliver timely and useful information. (3) Plans developed by the MOH show evidence of weak planning capacity. (4) Many important policy issues have not been addressed.

❖ *Deconcentration of resources* toward the first level of care is progressing.
However: (1) There are neither benchmarks against which annual performance by the districts is evaluated, nor a formula to assure funding equity. As a result, the allocation of resources is based on historical precedence rather than outputs, outcomes, or need. (2) Operating costs at the first and second levels of service remain highly dependent on user charges and external aid.

❖ *Decentralization:* The process has stalled because of controversy in both the legal and political arenas. Establishment of the Ghana Health Service has stalled because of unresolved issues between the DHMTs and the local government system regarding planning authority and financing responsibilities. Politically, the issue involves disagreements about responsibility for overall development and supervision of services at the local level.

❖ *Performance-based contracting:* Although the format for agreement between the MOH and the Mission hospitals was approved, and 21 out of the 43 hospitals met financial readiness criteria in 1998, no contracts between the government and hospitals were developed. Despite this, the government has continued to make payments to the Mission Hospitals.

❖ *Demand side issues:* Supply side aspects of service provision have been the primary focus, and few efforts have been made to gain an understanding of the determinants of utilization or of how to improve access for women and the poor.

OBSERVATIONS
AND POSSIBLE LESSONS

The Ghana Health Sector SWAP was the first SWAP in the social sector to encompass a whole sector, and it goes furthest in pooling resources and using government procedures.

(1) It is important for donors to avoid resentment for undue intervention in the Government's affairs in a sector approach. The donors should recognize that they do not determine decisions. The Government is in the driver's seat and does what it wants ultimately. Donors should react to what Government proposes rather than taking the initiative. SWAPs are possible if donors do not stick to their own vision or pet ideas, but see themselves much more as brokers and/or skeptics. The donor role is changing as the national policy capacity increases.

(2) It took longer than normal to prepare the SWAP for donor financing, largely because of the number and breadth of issues to be resolved and because of specific disagreements over the affordability and desirability of the capital program.

(3) SWAPs need a context in which the government is strong and has stability so that it can take the time to discuss and address the sectoral issues.

(4) Stability is also needed on the donor side to afford time to build up confidence among the donors themselves, and with the Government. SWAPs cannot be developed in a "stop and go" context.

(5) The Ghana Health SWAP grew out of circumstances that were almost unique. It cannot be transposed elsewhere. For example, the progress toward pooling of donor funds is built upon significant investments in financial management systems and supervision that may not exist elsewhere (Peters and Chao: 184).

(6) A SWAP does not have the security of a traditional project, where content and quantities are well defined in advance. Instead, the security must be implicit in the procedures by which decisions will be made during implementation.

(7) It took time to get implementation organized after the start of the program, including agreement on independent auditors, and the preparation of a procurement plan. Implementation issues were considered at the design stage but, understandably, they received less attention than agreements on policy, program content, and definition of indicators. It is important to recognize in advance the need for, and accelerate work on, key implementation activities.

(8) The annual system of reports, reviews, budget planning, and revisions in the program needs to be planned in detail. Terms of reference for the reviews, and joint responsibilities were determined in advance. They were changed several times before and during the reviews themselves. Similarly, the quarterly reports and budget systems were also designed ahead of time, and used before the project was effective. The importance of having worked out mechanisms and responsibilities is

underscored. It is very important to have a system in place by which views by all parties can be aired and disagreements resolved. In the end it is not so important that disputes and differences occur so long as a process of mutual consultation is in place and methods have been agreed in advance on how to resolve disputes and solve problems.[17]

(9) It is not enough to prepare a set of indicators by which to measure performance. A system must also be in place to collect the information, analyze and report on it. Even this is often not enough. There must be a place to conduct dialogue over the results. Health summits offer this venue. Bank staff found it highly stimulating to see various stakeholders (MOH HQ and regions, NGO and the minority representatives) discussing the review results.

(10) Under a sector-wide approach the donors need to keep in touch with all developments in the sector. It is easy to miss important topics, such as not looking sufficiently at the private sector—an acknowledged gap in the design of the HSSP. This has several implications: (a) a local technical presence may be necessary to keep the dialogue going; (b) more frequent missions may be needed; and (c) better capacity is needed by donors to analyze the issues and present alternatives, requiring different skills than heretofore has been the case with most donors – e.g., policy analysis and an ability to present and negotiate recommendations on policy issues.

(11) One observer stated, "Because of its national perspective and wide scope, the sector-wide program is less likely to promote participation at the local level and broaden ownership through the current implementation processes" (Annan: iii). However, ownership is actually determined by the type of reforms put into place. In this case, increased resources and authorities went to local levels, along with increased accountabilities and needs to involve users of health services locally.

(12) "Strong local leadership of the SWAP process is required, but this may initially involve a few committed actors. It is, however, essential for external partners to recognize early the need to progress from support to, and dialogue with, individuals and small groups to a wider institutional involvement that will ultimately build capacity for a larger group of professionals and provide greater scope for skills" (Annan, p. 28).

BIBLIOGRAPHY

Annan, Joe. 1999. "Ghana Health Sector-wide Programme: A Case Study." JSA Consultants, Ltd., Accra. Prepared for DAC I/CD Network and Policy Branch of CIDA, April 1999.

Decaillet, Francois. 1999. "Ghana: Health Sector Support Project—Back to Office Report." June 1, 1999.

Peters, David, and Shiyan Chao. 1998. "The Sector-Wide Approach in Health: What Is It? Where Is It Leading?" *International Journal of Health Planning and Management* 13: 177-190.

---

[8] Comments on this by project staff involved include the following: In hindsight, it would have been preferable not to air all disputes in a large open forum—this led to increased rigidity and some posturing that may have been worked out through other means. Instead of spending years designing a process for mutual consultation, it should be tried out. Good, willing people are more important than procedures. Instead of rewarding the elaboration of procedures, one should develop a system to reward people for solving problems.

Republic of Ghana. 1998. "Memorandum of Understanding: Ghana Health Sector Programme of Work." April 30.

Republic of Ghana. 1999. "Health Sector 5-Year Programme of Work 1997-2001: 1998 Review." Ministry of Health, Accra, April.

World Bank. 1997. "Memorandum and Recommendation of the President of the International Development Association to the Executive Directors on a Proposed Credit in the Amount Equivalent to SDR 25.1 Million to the Republic of Ghana for a Health Sector Program Support Project." Report No. P 7179 GH, September 25, 1997.

World Bank. 1997. "Staff Appraisal Report: Republic of Ghana Health Sector Support Program." Human Development III, Ghana Country Department, Report No. 16467-GH, September 25, 1997.

"Aide Memoire: Joint Ministry of Health—Health Partners Summit Meeting (May 5-7, 1999), Review of the 1998 Programme of Work." 7 May 1999.

TABLE 2
Progress in 20 Annual Performance Indicators

Indicator	Level	1996 Baseline			1997			1998		
					GOG	**DONOR**	**IGF**	**GOG**	**DONOR**	**IGF**
1. Percentage Government of Ghana recurrent budget spent on health.		7%			8.4%			8.6%		
2. a) Recurrent expenditure by level and source (ITEMS 2-5)		GOG	DONOR	IGF						
	Headquarters	28.1%			29%		2%	5%	27%	0%
	Tertiary institutions	31.5%			22%		30%	22%	4%	94%
	Regional	17.1%			15%		2%	13%	30%	0%
	District	23.3%			34%		66%	60%	39%	6%
2. b) Capital expenditure by level and source in % (items 7-9)	Headquarters				53%			25%	N/K	N/K
	Tertiary inst.				11%			20%	N/K	N/K
	Regional				34%			27%	N/K	N/K
	District				2%			28%	N/K	N/K
3. a) Percentage Budget and Management Centers with budget and plans.	Headquarters				47.6%			N/A		
	Teaching Hospitals				100%			N/A		
	Psychiatric Hospitals				100%			N/A		
	Reg. Health Admin.				100%			100%		
	Regional Hospitals				100%			100%		
	Health Training Inst.				89%			100%		
	District Health Admin.				100%			100%		
	District Hospitals				76%			98%		
	Sub-districts				63%			N/A		
3. b) Meeting readiness criteria:					57%			57%		
4. Percentage Budget and Management Centers with quarterly income and expenditure returns.		50%			63%			100%		
5. Contracts for mission hospitals, NGO and private service providers developed and in use.		Being developed as part of the performance monitoring system.			Memorandum of Understanding developed and consensus meeting held with Mission Hospitals.			None.		
6. Development of a single set of procurement procedures.	Goods	Bidding document developed.			Procurement unit (PU) set up.			PU Established Procurement Manual developed and adopted.		
	Civil works	Draft guidelines prepared.			Options appraisal applied to major capital projects.			In progress.		
	Technical assistance				Draft guidelines developed. List of TA procurement for 1998 prepared.			Standard Bidding Document completed List of TA for 1999 prepared.		

(continued on the next page)

71

TABLE 2 *(continued)*

Indicator		1996 Baseline	1997	1998
7. a) Completion of staffing establishments for BMCs.	Regional level BMCs	Estab. for tech staff completed.	100% completed.	100%
	Headquarters BMCs		80% subject to redefinition of Organigram	100%
	Statutory bodies		None completed. Process ongoing.	None completed. In progress
	Tertiary level BMCs		40% completed. New BMCs yet to be done.	80%
7. b) Percentage BMCs with 90% to 105% staffing establishment filled.	Regional level BMCs			N/A
	Headquarters BMCs Statutory bodies			100%
	Tertiary level BMCs			N/A
8. Percentage districts with communicable disease surveillance reports.	Greater Accra		60%	100%
	Eastern Region		80%	100%
	Central region		70%	100%
	Western Region		60%	80%
	Volta Region		80%	75%
	Ashanti Region		70%	100%
	Brong Ahafo Reg.		90%	100%
	Northern Region		80%	N/K
	Upper East Reg.		100%	100%
	Upper West R.		100%	100%

9. Outpatient visits	REGION	TOTAL	MALE	FEMALE	TOTAL	MALE	FEMALE	TOTAL	MALE	FEMALE
	Ashanti	1390704	643417	747287	1334441	615292	719149	1399110	N/A	N/A
	Brong Ahafo	830982	384218	446764	970335	447423	522912	923773	N/A	N/A
	Central	275262	148512	127740	337401	160072	177329	410344	N/A	N/A
	Eastern	758755	320184		713993	292736	438571	739894	N/A	N/A
	Greater Accra	1258041	504449	753592	1277251	538900	738351	1215489	N/A	N/A
	Northern	273563	143437	130126	364480	178400	186080	364649	N/A	N/A
	Upper East	297905	142560	155345	173937	85184	88753	194338	N/A	N/A
	Upper West	130471	68639	61832	152810	79263	73547	161383		
	Volta	530604	235267	295337	565485	240150	325338	658280	N/A	N/A
	Western	603398	277844	325554	656637	304560	352077	686102	N/A	N/A
	National	6350675	2868527	3482148	6546773	2941980	3604793	6753363	N/A	N/A
OPD visits per year		0.36			0.36			0.35		

10. a) Hospital admissions	LEVEL	PUBLIC	Male / female	PUBLIC	Male / female	PUBLIC	Male	Female
	Teaching Hospital	80979		92528		91987	N/A	N/A
	Regional Hospital and District hospitals	354688		392531		389337	N/A	N/A
Per 1000 pop		25.0		26.5		25.5		

Indicator		1996 Baseline	1997	1998
10. b) Bed occupancy	**LEVEL**	**PUBLIC**	**PUBLIC**	**PUBLIC**
	Teaching Hospital	90.8%	91.3%	91.7%
	Regional Hospital	70.1%	70.8%	71.5%
	District hospitals	65.2%	67.2%	71.3%
10. c) Average	Teaching Hospital	8.5	8.2	7.5
	Regional Hospital	7.4	7.2	6.3
	District hospitals	7.8	7.5	5.2
11. EPI coverage		DPT3 51.4%	59.6%	67.5%
		OPV3 53.2%	58.5%	67.5%
12. Family planning – Couple years protection (% CYPs of no. WIFA)		251,762 (6.0%)	264,412 (7.7%)	346,523 (9,2%)
13. Percentage children using bednets		Less than 1%	Less than 1%	Less than 1%
14. Condom sales		2,230,900	2,126,171	2,105,716
15. Percentage tracer drug availability/essential drugs stocked at the district level		(80%)	(86.8%)	CMS 87% RMS: 92% DMS: 90% Health Facility: 83%
16. Medical equipment performance index		60%	70%	N/K
17. Average cost per inpatient day	District hospital		¢27,500	¢14,347
	Regional hosp.		¢33,000	¢35, 848
	Tertiary hospital			¢39, 009

18. Amount spent on exemptions by exemption category	**CATEGORY**	**1996**	**1997**	**1998**
	Paupers	N/A	N/A	¢ 390 m.
	Antenatal Services		¢2.6b	¢ 1,515 m.
	Aged (over 70)		¢0.7b	¢ 429 m.
	Children (under 5)		—	¢ 54 m.
	Psychiatry/Leprosy		¢2.8b	N/A
	Emergency cases			¢ 153 m.
	Others		¢ 0.4b	¢ 191m.

19. Number of outreach clinics by region (average number of sites per health facility) Absolute number of outreach sites, by year: 1996 . . . . 6,677 1997 . . . . 7,436 1998 10,249	Ashanti Region	5	5	
	Brong Ahafo Reg.	6	6	7.6
	Central Region	10	10	14.2
	Eastern Region	8	9	5.3
	Greater Accra	9	9	16.2
	Northern Region	11	11	14.7
	Upper East Reg.	5	7	7.0
	Upper West Reg.	8	9	11.9
	Volta Region	5	8	17.9
	Western Region	6	7	9.2
	National (average)	7	7.7	11.1

20. Percentage district, regional, and teaching hospitals reporting on patient satisfaction.	Teaching Hospital	0%	0%	0%
	Regional Hospital	22%	33.3%	56%
	District Hospital	13%	33%	10%

TABLE 3
949 – Ghana, Health SCTR Support
Project Status Report Date: **6/11/99**

Region:	AFR	Country:	GHANA			Sector:	HH	Lending Instr:	SIL
Prg Obj Cat:	PA	EA Cat:	C	PTI?	N	NGO?	Y	Resettlement?	N

LOAN INFORMATION

Agree Type	L/C/G No.	Orig Amt	Rev'd Amt	Currency Indicator	Prod Line	Signing Date	Effective Date	Suppl Prj ID
IDA	29940	25.10 (SDR)			PE	4/3/98	6/18/98	

Total Original Amount (SDR):	25.10	Total Revised Amount (SDR):	0.00

COFINANCING INFORMATION

Agency	Board Amount ($M)	Current Amount ($M)
ADF		4.40
BADEA		4.50
CIDA		0.20
DANIDA		30.10
DIGIS		9.60
EU-EC		9.00
GTZ		4.50
JICA		0.90
ODA		47.00
OPEC-SF		5.00
PRIVATE		77.00
SAUDI F		2.30
UNFPA		10.00
UNICEF		10.00
USAID		12.00
WHO		4.30
Total	0.00	230.80

Guarantee Type:		Guarantee Amount ($M):	

This form is part of: **Portfolio status update**
Read together with:

( ) Aide-memoire	Mission End Date:	5/13/99	This Form PSR Date:	6/11/99
( ) BTO memo of:	Months since last mission:	9	Last Form PSR Date:	2/3/99
( ) Follow-up letter of:	Next mission planned:	9/15/99		

SUPERVISION EFFORT	Total Staff-Weeks	Total $000	Field Staff-Weeks	Field $000	As of 6/11/99
Current FY - Planned	58.40	121.84			
Current FY - Actual	55.68	127.37	0.00	0.00	
Board through preceding FY	16.88	75.65	0.00	0.00	
Total Actual	72.56	203.02	0.00	0.00	

UPI No.	Mission Member	Division	No. of Fld Days	Role or Specialization	Previous Mission
66828	DECAILLET	AFTH3	12.0	PUBLIC HEALTH, TTL	Y

Senegal Health Case Study[1]
Integrated Health Sector Development Program (IHSDP)

BACKGROUND

IDA financed a multi-sectoral human resources development project (PDRH1) in 1991 for US$35 million. The health component, implemented in three regions, highlighted the need for the consideration of human resource management issues in the context of civil service reform, and the importance of building the capacity of the central administration in the context of decentralization. The impact of change initiated under the PDRH1 project and the sectoral studies it helped finance, enhanced the Bank's policy dialogue with Government on health sector development. It also paved the way for significant reforms in health financing and the development of a comprehensive framework for improving health system management, decentralized management, and the promotion of health insurance. Sectoral studies under PDRH1 raised four critical issues for the health sector: (1) inadequate and inequitable financing of curative care; (2) low efficiency in the use of resources by public sector health facilities; (3) low utilization and access to health care and family planning services; and (4) inadequate human resources and lack of effective human resource development in the sector.

The background to the SIP is also characterized by a proliferation of health projects financed by a multitude of donors. All parties realized that this fragmented approach was not conducive to the development of the sector as a whole. Government was not in a position to coordinate the activities of all donors. There was no single policy or vision for the sector. The Government was ready to adopt a sector-wide approach and willing to take the lead in its development.

SWAP DESIGN

Basic data: Kind of lending instrument: Sector Investment Loan (SIL). The elapsed time for program development was 85.7 weeks (from Concept Review to Decision Meeting). The time between appraisal and Board presentation was 14.9 weeks (see attached data sheet).

Rationale for the SWAP: The main impetus for the SWAP was the lack of performance and impact on sector-wide issues from the classic project approach. The country had been divided into a mosaic of small projects (over 20 projects) that did not add up to an impact on overall sectoral issues. There was a general recognition that many of the issues in the sector were system-wide (such as administration, human resources, financial sustainability) and could not be addressed in an insular, piecemeal fashion.

---

[1] Based on an interview with Mr. Anwar Bach-Baouab, Task Team Leader, and the Staff Appraisal Report, No. 16756-SE, August 8, 1997.

"The issues facing the sector are systemic and require a broader systemic response" (SAR, p. 17). As further stated in the SAR, "The issue of a traditional investment project versus a broader sectoral investment program was thoroughly discussed with Government and donor agencies during the program identification and preparation stages. The decision to move forward with a sector approach is based on: (a) the willingness of donors to participate in a sector investment program and support implementation of the Government development plan, and (b) commitment of the Government to define a long-term policy framework which addresses all key issues of health financing, efficiency and sustainability. In addition, implementation of the health reform agenda initiated in 1991 was well sustained during the past five years. … This has laid the foundation for a comprehensive reform of the health sector involving all major stakeholders" (pp. 15–16).

SWAP characteristics: The program is sector-wide in scope; it is based on an agreed sector policy and strategy; it is founded on an agreed expenditure program; the Government clearly has leadership of the process; all main donors have agreed to the program and to finance a share of its costs.

Preconditions: Besides a favorable macroeconomic environment, the following pre-conditions were met for starting to develop a sector-wide approach: (1) Government commitment and willingness to take leadership; (2) donor commitment to the sector-wide approach; (3) clear strategic vision by the Ministry of Health; and (4) a minimum institutional capacity as indicated by the implementation of previous projects.

Definition of the sector: The Health Sector Program is not limited to any aspects but encompasses the overall health system: primary, secondary, and tertiary health care. It focuses on two major generic issues for the sector: human resource development and health sector financing. Thus, the "sector" is congruent with the existing management organization for planning and budgeting.

Program leadership: The Ministry of Health (MOH) led the process of program development. One of the successes in the operation was the will-ingness of the Ministry of Finance to work hand in hand with the MOH in designing the program, which augured well for success in program implementation. The Ministries of Health and Finance established a National Task Force composed of highly motivated members from both ministries. This Task Force was the driving force behind program design. Technical support was provided by donors during the program design process. Donors were given the opportunity to review and comment on draft versions of the program documents.

Donor coordination: The European Union (EU) was the lead agency for donor coordination. One of the major elements for the success of the program was that the Bank did not take the lead among donors. The Bank was not seen as driving the process. The EU convened regular monthly donors meetings and maintained official correspondence with the Government. In contrast with the past, a systematic sharing of information was achieved. Also, donors made an effort to associate other donor partners in the program so as to work in a complementary manner.

Program development: (1) The National Task Force first agreed on an action plan for the design of the program. (2) The second step was to undertake a series of studies on the assessment of human resources, health financing, hospital reform, assessment of primary health care, and cost recovery. Donor funds were readily available to finance these studies. (3) Third, based on the findings the Task Force developed a "Long-Term Strategic Vision for Health Development." (4) Fourth, the Task Force then developed a 10-year National Health Plan, which identified critical priorities and implementation mechanisms with technical support from multilateral and bilateral donors and involving extensive consultations with stakeholders. Government ownership of the design process was strong, with MOH being the driving force behind the process. (5) The long-term plan then led to the preparation of a "Five-Year Action Plan" that spelled out immediate priorities and investment requirements. (6) The Ministers of Health and Finance convened a roundtable of donors at which the Plan was reviewed by donors and pledges were made for the financing of the Plan. This resulted in a well-conceived financing plan, including both national and external sources. (7) Program appraisal came right after the roundtable. Key program documents (strategic framework /long-term plan /and medium-term expenditure program) were reviewed and commented on by donors at regular intervals in the program design process and officially endorsed at the roundtable. In the process as a whole there were few disagreements of a substantive nature. Differences centered mainly on administrative and financial procedures.

Level of sector analysis: The prior IDA project, PDRH1 (Human Resources Development Project) financed several sector studies that formed the basis for the IHSDP. In addition, in the design of the Program new studies were carried out in the areas of health financing, institutional development, hospital reform, reproductive health, and human resources development. These were also financed relatively quickly under the ongoing operation, which greatly facilitated program design.

Institutional capacity: International experts were employed during program design to assess the organization, structure, and administration of the health system. Recommendations led to the adoption of an institution development plan and a program of reform, including a plan for restructuring the Ministry of Health. In addition, the Program emphasizes measures for staff recruitment and training at the district level.

Stakeholder consultation: Program development followed a highly participatory approach. The views of NGOs, civil society, associations of physicians, and pharmacists and different ministries were solicited through a series of workshops and debates on the national health plan. This achieved a wide consensus on the contents when the final plans were prepared. The same was true for the development of the Five-Year Action Plan. In the end there were no major disagreements on policies or strategies.

THE IHSDP PROGRAM

Aims and content: The IHSDP seeks to improve the quality, access, and sustainability of health delivery systems as a means to improve the health status of the population and accelerate transition toward slower population growth. The Program will (1) expand access to primary health care and referral services to the majority of the population; (2) improve the quality, efficiency, and effectiveness of health care provision including reproductive health information and services, and (3) strengthen the MOH institutional capacity to efficiently organize, monitor, and evaluate health services. In particular, the Program includes hospital reform, restructuring of the Ministry of Health, decentralization of planning and management of health services to districts, and a comprehensive training plan for health staff.

Financing: The discussions on the Five-Year Action Plan and pledging, by donors yielded a good overall financing plan. During pledging, coverage of at least the first two years of the program was stressed. The third and fourth year of implementation would be taken into account later. This introduced flexibility in the financing. Some donors could pledge now or later for future years of the program. The total cost of the five-year program was estimated at about $410 million, including both investment and recurrent expenditures. External donors were expected to finance about 30% of the total cost and—within this —the IDA Credit of US$50 million would finance about 12% of the total cost. Fourteen donors will participate in funding the program.[2] The Bank is the donor of last resort. At appraisal the amount of the Credit was determined on the basis of the size of the expected gap in program financing. The Bank iden-

---

[2] AfDB, the EU, IDB, NDF, JICA, KFW, the Kingdom of Belgium, the French Cooperation Agency, the Netherlands Cooperation, Taiwan, USAID, Unicef, UNFPA, and IDA.

tified the program elements that were not taken by other donors in the first two years and specified those for its initial financing. The balance (about 61%) of the Credit proceeds are left unallocated to allow flexibility for adjustment in years three to five of program implementation. The Bank will pick up the financing of components left after other donors have chosen, provided the Bank is satisfied that all programs of high priority are being financed.

Procurement: Procurement under the program is rather similar to that under a traditional project, but donors agreed on a common procurement plan that identified their respective input and timing.

Financial flows and disbursements: Considerable discussion took place among the donors during Program design about "basket funding", or the pooling of resources. It was clear from earlier SIPs in the health sector (Zambia, Ghana) that pooling resources was problematic. Therefore in the case of Senegal it was decided to adopt a flexible approach. Funds are not forced into a single basket. Basket funding was included at the district level for recurrent expenditures, with donors making their contribution into a single district account using advances of funds or reimbursement mechanisms. However, the bulk of the financing is parallel funding. The donors contribute to common accounts, but arrangements have been made so that each donor input can be identified and disbursements are kept separate for accounting purposes. The process reportedly has worked well and has enabled funds to be channeled to districts. The operation is regarded as a first generation of SWAPs, a step toward transition to eventual budgetary assistance. Before that occurs, however, considerable strengthening will be needed in the Government's administrative and management procedures to enable a majority of donors to use them.

Risks and dangers: There are no special risks associated with this SWAP in terms of approach. The four risks mentioned in the SAR are: (1) slower than expected change in fertility; (2) continuation of weak implementation capacity at the MOH compounded by difficulties in staff recruitment and retention in the regions; (3) difficulties in the devolution of health

administration to local government; and (4) unforeseen economic difficulties slowing or reversing increases in health expenditures.

Conditionality: Very few conditions are attached to the IDA credit. The process of Program design led to widespread consensus and commitment to the reforms adopted in the Program. Specific assurances included: (a) actions to increase overall health expenditures to 8.2% of total public expenditures by 2002; (b) financing of the Program in accordance with the agreed financing plan; (c) submission of work programs and budgets at least three months before the joint annual review; and (d) submission of progress reports on agreed performance indicators and use of funds before the joint annual reviews (SAR, p. 47). Conditions, thus, focus mainly on the process for annual review and adjustment of the program. This review process was designed to be flexible, with a self-adjusting process, so that allocations could be adjusted each year in relation to performance and prevailing conditions. No separate remedies were considered necessary.

SWAP IMPLEMENTATION

Organization for implementation: The MOH is responsible for overall implementation of the Program, through its Directorate of General Administration, Finance and Equipment (DAGE) and Technical Divisions. A special Support Unit (SSU) was created at the cabinet level within the MOH to oversee the management of resources provided under the Program.

Modus operandi: As stated in the SAR, "the Sectoral Investment Program initiative adopted for the IHSDP emphasizes a continuing policy dialogue and phased funding, based on yearly operational plans, ... eligibility criteria for program resources and sector-wide performance indicators. ... This would be achieved through joint Government/Donors annual implementation reviews" (Summary). The joint annual reviews are the key element in the implementation process. "The program will be implemented through a series of joint annual agreements based on assessment of previous years performance and operational plans and budgets based on priorities and established eligibility criteria for access to program funding. This procedure will allow Government, IDA and other financing institutions to adjust to changing conditions and performance thereby building in a higher level of flexibility which will allow for more realistic planning on a year by year basis" (SAR, p. 21). Plans call for five such annual agreements, each covering one fiscal year from 1998 to 2002. Each will summarize the detailed individual agreement for specific categories of expenditure. Annual reviews are timed to coincide with the Government's fiscal year. Monitoring and information systems, common for all donors, are a key to the success of annual reviews. Two sets of data are collected: (a) Critical performance benchmarks: for the first two years these include placement of program management staff, acceptable allocations to each expenditure category, levels of disbursement, recruitment and training of staff, and having MIS in place in all districts. (b) Performance indicators for districts include: increase in the use of health facilities, proportion of children vaccinated, increases in prenatal consultations, and increases in contraceptive prevalence.

Implementation experience: Two mid-year reviews and one annual meeting have been held with strong Government/Donors/Stakeholders participation. The experience thus far has revealed certain weaknesses. First, the management information system is not yet satisfactory. Data are not flowing from the regions to the central region. In part this is the result of a "greve du Zele", where health staff in the regions strike by withholding data. This has required ad hoc studies to gather data on program performance in the regions. Other implementation problems have resulted from difficulties on the part of central MOH authorities to delegate functions to regional offices. The decentralization has been agreed to in principle, but effective mechanisms to manage the relationship between elected bodies and the deconcentrated sectoral entities have not yet become fully operational. Sometimes this is being resisted

in practice. This has slowed the overall implementation of the Program. Another implementation issue, not surprisingly, is the limited implementation capacity at district levels. The Program includes assistance for recruitment and training of staff, but the impact has not been immediately felt at the district level.

OUTCOMES SO FAR

Main achievements: So far the successes include: (1) the political commitment and Government ownership for the overall policies, strategies and program; (2) donor cohesiveness and shared approaches; (3) an agreed strategic vision and framework that addresses critical issues; (4) a comprehensive, system-wide, and national approach rather than the focus on small elements of the system; (5) accomplishment of a participatory approach, including the signing of six major contracts with NGOs for the implementation of health service delivery; and (6) adoption of a common financing, implementation, and procurement plan by the donors and the use of common indicators, supervision, and reporting procedures.

LESSONS

The following lessons should be noted:

(1) The Bank should strive to step away from the lead role in program design to encourage complementarity among donors and to promote ownership.

(2) Set the parameters of the design process at an early stage in terms of who is in charge, the role of each agency, how donor collaboration will be achieved, and participation by stakeholders.

(3) Confirm that the five criteria or preconditions mentioned above are met, or likely to be met in the early stages of program development before starting on the process.

(4) Basket funding, or pooling of resources, is not necessary at first. A "transition SWAP" can be designed that allows donors to contribute funds in accordance with their own procedures that can be accounted for separately, while working on a common objective of strengthening government procedures that could be used by all parties at a later stage.

(5) It is important for the Bank to show some flexibility in order to play its role as donor of last resort and to cover any financing gaps that might emerge during program implementation.

TABLE 1
2369 – Senegal Integr. Health S. Dev.
Project Status Report Date: **6/22/99**

Region:	AFR	Country:	SENEGAL			Sector:	HH	Lending Instr:	SIL
Prg Obj Cat:	PA	EA Cat:	C	PTI?	Y	NGO?	Y	Resettlement?	N

LOAN INFORMATION

Agree Type	L/C/G No.	Orig Amt	Rev'd Amt	Currency Indicator	Prod Line	Signing Date	Effective Date	Suppl Prj ID
IDA	29850	35.90 (SDR)			PE	9/15/97	2/2/98	

Total Original Amount (SDR):	35.90	Total Revised Amount (SDR):	0.00

COFINANCING INFORMATION

Agency	Board Amount ($M)	Current Amount ($M)
AFDB	10.00	10.00
BEL	2.00	2.00
EU-EC	14.00	14.00
FAC	1.00	0.00
FPPI	4.00	4.00
FRA		1.00
GTZ	3.00	3.00
ISLAMIC	5.00	5.00
ITA	3.00	3.00
KFW	3.00	3.00
NDF	5.00	5.00
NET	4.00	4.00
UNICEF	5.00	5.00
Total	59.00	59.00

Guarantee Type:	Guarantee Amount ($M):

This form is part of: **Supervision Mission**
Read together with:

( ) Aide-memoire	Mission End Date:	6/4/99	This Form PSR Date:	6/22/99
( ) BTO memo of:	Months since last mission:	8	Last Form PSR Date:	12/14/98
( ) Follow-up letter of: 6/4/99	Next mission planned:	10/18/99		

SUPERVISION EFFORT	Total Staff-Weeks	Total $000	Field Staff-Weeks	Field $000	As of 6/22/99
Current FY - Planned	27.50	70.85			
Current FY - Actual	37.38	87.78	0.00	0.00	
Board through preceding FY	21.10	65.85	0.00	0.00	
Total Actual	58.48	153.63	0.00	0.00	

UPI No.	Mission Member	Division	No. of Fld Days	Role or Specialization	Previous Mission
185252	SY	AFMSN	20.0	HNP OPERATION SPEC.	Y
95309	THEUNYNCK	AFTH2	2.0	IMPL. SPEC	Y
185252	SY	AFTH2	20.0	HNP CLUSTER LEADER	Y

Zambia Health Case Study[1]
Health Sector Support Project (HSSP)

BACKGROUND

Since independence the Government had used its international borrowing capacity to support levels of consumption in the public sector that proved unproductive and unsustainable as its wealth— dependent on copper prices—declined. At the time of initial project design, Zambia suffered from excessive public sector dominance, a decline of nearly 50% in per capita income since 1975, and a dramatic increase in poverty. Funding cuts in all social sectors during the economic crisis of the 1980s had led to several dilapidation of health infrastructure. The health sector was overwhelmed as population growth, combined with increasing incidences of diseases, such as AIDS and malaria, raised demands for basic health care. Infant mortality rates rose, the prevalence of malnutrition increased, and vaccination rates for children fell. Access to health facilities, the quality of services, and the availability of drugs and supplies varied widely. Health staff were concentrated in urban hospitals (80 percent of all physicians) while health facilities in rural areas with 60% of the population remained understaffed.

The commitment to change was established in November 1991 when a new government was elected on a platform of adjustment and policy reform. The rehabilitation and reform of social service delivery was a key area of concern in Zambia's adjustment program and development strategy. Government commitment to improving health services had been evidenced by increased allocations to health (from 6% of the budget to 13% in 1994/5/6). Its commitment to reform was manifested in the 1991 National Health Policy paper which outlined the government's aims for reforming the health sector in order to provide Zambians with "equity of access to cost-effective quality health care as close to the family as possible."

SECTOR PROGRAM DESIGN

Lending Instrument: The project is supported by a Sector Investment and Maintenance Loan (SIM). In fact, it is a Sector Investment Program (SIP), one of the first to have been financed in the social sector in Africa. The government took the lead in preparing a common framework under which donors to the sector, including IDA, could provide support. The main components of the SIP approach were:

* ❖ The development of a single, comprehensive strategic framework that could be agreed on by all "Cooperating Partners".

---

[1] Based on interviews with Ms. Julie McLaughlin, former Task Team Leader, and the sources listed in the bibliography at the end of the case.

❖ An annual implementation plan and annual comprehensive budget for the investment and operating costs of the sector. Donors were asked to structure their support to meet those financing needs that could not be met by government – primarily investment costs.

❖ Joint implementation procedures – accounting, disbursement, reporting, monitoring, and evaluation.

Rationale for the sector program: One of the reasons a sector program was undertaken was the government's comprehensive vision of the sector. This included innovative approaches including a shift toward primary from tertiary care and decentralization to districts. A second reason is that the Bank wanted to support donor-initiated reforms. As stated in the SAR, "There is no practical alternatives to the proposed sector approach, as a traditional investment project would destroy the Government-led process of reforms…" (SAR, p. 30). Third, although the Bank had no previous projects and direct experience with lending for health in Zambia, experience in other countries demonstrated the need for more comprehensive and integrated involvement in the health sector to ensure sustainable development impact (SAR, p. 32). One reason was that projects typically have gaps in financing that leave critical inputs underfinanced. Another reason was the "replacement mentality" where project funds allow government funds to be used for other, less priority, purposes, i.e., "fungability."

Preconditions: Macroeconomic stability was cited later as a condition for starting a sector-wide approach in Zambia, but those developing the project focused on sector-specific issues dealing with reform. The impetus of the reform was the government commitment and efforts to reform the health system along lines endorsed by the Bank. In effect, this was the precondition that led to the development of the sector program. Other considerations were secondary.

Definition of the sector: The sector includes all things for which the Ministry of Health is responsible. The definition is thus comprehensive,[2] including central, district and local levels – as well as all programs undertaken by the Ministry. There were no other agencies of government explicitly responsible for health.

Program leadership: The impetus for reforms came clearly from the government. Zambian officials clearly were driving the health sector reforms and program development. In the run-up to the first national election in 1991, the eventual party that won prepared a manifesto on health reform. The person who wrote the party manifesto on health became the Deputy Minister of Health. Shortly thereafter the government approached the Bank informally about support for the program. The Bank found the program innovative and wanted to respond in an innovative manner. There was no model for supporting a sector-wide program. The program design was developed almost exclusively by the government (specifically the Deputy Minister of Health and the chief health planner), with donor involvement increasingly only later in the process. As the Task Team Leader said, "IDA jumped on a moving train."

Donor coordination: The government took the initiative to get donors interested in the program. Initially IDA, the WHO, and UNICEF were the agencies most interested. DANIDA was the first bilateral participating in preparation, followed by the Swedes, Dutch, and British. IDA instigated donor coordination, but it was performed by the government. The government called and hosted all the donor meetings and missions.

Program development: The first step in program development was taken by Zambian officials in the preparation of the National Health Policy paper in

---

[2] Later, there was a mistaken impression in some quarters that the sector program was not in fact sector-wide and dealt only with districts (perhaps because pooled financing was limited to district grants).

1991 based on the party manifest. The second step was the preparation of the Strategic Plan during 1992–93 with Bank assistance. The adoption of a sector-wide approach compelled the Bank to become involved in the national planning of comprehensive health care reform rather than focusing on pieces of the reform process, the traditional project approach. As an integral part of this work a Bank mission introduced a health planning framework to the Ministry of Health in May 1993. The tangible output that was catalyzed by this planning process was the Strategic Plan for health reform, which details plans for how the new health system will operate, what inputs it requires, and how the Ministry intends to transform the existing system into the new one envisaged. In preparing the Strategic Plan the Ministry of Health formed committees around each component of the reforms. They: (1) undertook a critical assessment of health needs, identifying financial, physical, human, and academic resources and considering the stakeholders in the process; (2) defined a new set of health system standards—on the basis of equity and affordability principles— through packaging cost-effective health care; (3) identified requisite inputs and management support by level of institution and its anticipated workload; (4) estimated consequent costs by types of expenditure; (5) identified a health financing strategy to cover these costs, including ministry budget, private expenditures, and external donor support; and (6) committed the government to monitoring the progress of implementation and the impact of reform on target beneficiaries (SAR, pp. 6-7). The Bank subsequently assisted the development of policies regarding the financing of a minimum package of cost-effective health services, and determining how private financing might increase resources available to finance essential services. However, the Bank had little influence on the basic policy decisions (decentralization, charging user fees, delinking health staff from the civil service) as these decisions were rooted in the earlier Health Policy. The third step was appraisal in 1994 jointly by all interested donors. The government made a series of presentations about the program to donors. The mission appraised the

comprehensive health sector strategy, the budget envelope, decentralization, and the government's commitment to delivering an essential package of care. During the appraisal, several interest groups lobbied to increase the list of deliverables and the Zambian officials realized they would be in trouble if they tried to please everyone. This led to the adoption and use of cost-effectiveness analysis to determine what services to deliver. The appraisal focused on processes—the structural, legal, organization, and management of the delivery of a package of health services, rather than on traditional "programs", such as immunization or AIDS. In the sector support model for financing, project preparation and appraisal were focused on the nature of the apex institution's involvement and the *processes* by which specific investment items would be identified during implementation. In the end there was a lot of trial and error. The government minister supported the trial of different elements and allowed failure.

Level of sector analysis: The Bank had in its possession several earlier studies on sectoral issues from the late 1980s from the development of a health project that had never materialized. (In fact, a health mission was in the field working on the project when the Bank abruptly stopped its operations in Zambia and withdrew representation.) However, these were somewhat dated, and were not relevant to the comprehensive program. Some new studies were done on specific topics in preparation of the Strategic Plan, but much needed sector analysis was done after Credit commitment. For example, the expenditure review was done after effectiveness. After effectiveness, analytical work was done on human resource issues and "burden of disease" issues, and work continued on the definition of an effective minimum package of goods and services. In effect, the initial policies and plans—while generally found to be acceptable through appraisal—had been prepared without sufficient analytical background. The specific gaps were then filled during implementation. In effect, the Bank went to the Board in the midst of preparation without all the details. Since it was a process, it was felt that completion of preparation did not matter so much as donor commitment to the reform process and the agreed framework and objectives.

Institutional capacity: Institutional capacity was not analyzed rigorously in advance, and in retrospect may have been one of the weaker elements of program preparation. DANIDA was working on financial management and information systems and the Bank relied on that work. Even the Program Coordinator had to be trained on the job. The project launch was not particularly well thought through. In a way, the enthusiasm and commitment of Zambian officials for the reform program compensated for the initial lack of capacity to manage the program. The program was fortunate to have competent people involved and things went well initially for three years because of this.

Stakeholder consultation: Stakeholder consultation was done effectively. Many consultative meetings were held with district staff. The scope of consultation was relatively narrow initially, mainly focused on district public health providers. Gradually the "net" widened, in part with the encouragement of donors, to include hospital boards, private health providers, the few local NGOs that existed, and parastatal organizations (pharmaceutical company, mines). A deliberate decision was made to leave out central program managers (e.g., TB, AIDS, nutrition) from the initial consultation process because the reform was attempting to overcome the vertical "empires" such programs entailed. This was later regretted and rectified.

THE PROGRAM

Objectives, strategy, and content: The IDA project supports the government's health reform program with a view to improving access to, and the quality of, a national package of essential health services in a decentralized health care delivery system. This reform program was explained in the Strategic Plan and was agreed on with a core group of donors. IDA financing fits with the national health reform program, financing a slice of each of the three national budgets (investment, policy devel-

opment, and recurrent) based on annual agreements. The exact mix of financing would be determined on an annual basis, but with a three-year rolling program.

The Credit was divided into three major components, including (a) support for operations research and policy development (an estimated 3% of Credit proceeds); (b) investment program support (95%) and incremental recurrent budget support (1%); and (c) external monitoring and evaluation (1%), including beneficiary assessments and auditing. The overall investment program was to be a consolidation of investment programs prepared by individual districts, hospital boards, and the central MOH. It included three elements: (i) infrastructure and equipment, including "transparent criteria and standards ... in the Strategic Plan to enable the Health Boards to qualify for supplementary assistance and supervision" (SAR, p. 20); (ii) capacity building to improve planning and implementation skills at the various levels in the areas of clinical competence, corporate planning and management, monitoring and supervision; and (iii) supplies to ensure a regular supply of essential drugs and materials for the health service to function effectively.

Modus operandi: A detailed determination of components to be financed would be the outcome of a district planning process, a consolidation of individual plans prepared by districts and hospital boards. Thus, a "bottom-up" planning process is one of the key methods for the implementation of the program. These were not investment plans, but operational plans for non-personnel non-pharmaceutical recurrent costs, e.g., plans to increase immunization through improving the cold chain. Training seminars were provided for district staff in how to prepare plans. The center gave guidelines to the districts and seven referral hospital boards for how grant funds could be spent, such as limits on spending for certain items – for example, no more than a certain percentage on repairs, allowances, or fuel. The plans included the submission of a set of targets. If the plans were accepted, the district would receive a per capita allocation weighted in favor of poverty and rural areas. The criteria for evaluating the plans included consistency with national goals and the adequacy of specific programs proposed. Guidelines evolved and were developed further each year. They reflected emerging priorities and desired directions and strategies.

In traditional investment projects, the preparation and appraisal process focus on reviewing and planning the specific items (such as infrastructure or support systems) slated for financing. In this case, the project supports the government in ongoing development of policy and its operationalization, even as reforms are proceeding. Therefore specific items are being identified throughout the implementation of the project. The mechanism for identifying priorities and agreeing on budgets is the semiannual review. These reviews alternately assess progress in meeting previous agreements (April) and plans for the coming year (October). The April review covered the implementation of the entire health reform program as detailed in the Strategic Plan, not simply the components supported through donor, or IDA financing, and includes assessments of both finances and programs. The October review considered the annual update of the Strategic Plan as prepared by the Ministry of Health. It includes a rough, rolling two-year investment program, an annual recurrent cost budget, and identification of areas for which donor support is sought. At the same time, the Ministry presents an annual implementation plan with investment and recurrent cost budgets. Donor commitments are sought for the next year. Each donor then bilaterally structures its support on the basis of the documents and agreements.

The Planning and Management Unit (PMU) of the Ministry of Health, an existing unit that coordinates all donor-financed investment in the sector, was initially responsible for program oversight and management (all MOH-implemented). Subsequently, as the Central Board of Health (CBOH) was formed, the CBOH assumed responsibility for the bulk of oversight and management, but the MOH retained authority over implementation.

The development of common implementation procedures has received attention. DANIDA financed work aimed at developing joint government/donor accounting, reporting, and disbursement systems. The aim was to reduce demands for individual donor financial reports and facilitate an evolution toward a single "basket" account for the financing of the health sector. In an effort to better institutionalize monitoring and evaluation activities and reduce the demand on ministry program staff, a system of quarterly and annual joint reviews helps incorporate reporting and review requirements for all Cooperating Partners, and aims to supersede eventually the previous pattern of specific reviews by individual donors.

Financing: The total program cost was estimated at $537 million from 1995 to 1998. The Government was to finance $340 million (63%), IDA $56 million (10%), and other donors[3] $141 million (26%). No allowance was made for contingencies. "The number a size of activities would be revised to fit within the existing financing framework" (SAR, p. 34). A detailed determination of the investment items could not be made up front as this depended on the outcome of the district planning process, i.e., bottom-up planning, and annual agreement on the investment plan and recurrent budget. It was agreed that IDA would remain the "lender of last resort" by supporting those elements of an agreed-upon program for which no other donor funding could be identified. Some $6.3 million (11.3%) of the Credit proceeds were unallocated.

Risks and dangers: Abandonment of the health reforms was explicitly recognized in the appraisal report as a clear project risk, but it was felt that the risk had been minimized by adjustment credits. Another risk would be "internal political change." However, the SAR states: "Such change has already been weathered during the project preparation process.

---

[3] ODA, SIDA, DANIDA, The Netherlands, UNICEF.

The broad-based support and momentum for health reforms, both within the MOH and in districts across the country, would make it difficult for a different government or a different minister to annul what is already in the pipeline" (SAR, p. 41). Reference was also made to a risk that implementation of the Strategic Plan would be stalled on "process issues" without making impact on services and beneficiaries. It was assumed that lack of progress in making progress would be addressed in an acceptable manner within the annual review and planning process and the next year's plan of action (SAR, p. 42). A final risk noted was that donors may not agree to use common procedures and some would continue to provide aid with conditions that were not compatible with the agreed Strategic Plan. Continued dialogue among the donors and government, it was assumed, would minimize this risk.

Conditions: The IDA Credit came with relatively few conditions. A condition of effectiveness was the full financing of the investment program and budget for 1995. Conditions of disbursement were (i) acceptable standard architectural designs for district level facilities, and (ii) disbursement of $10 million on district facilities before any disbursement on central and regional facilities. The other conditions specified that implementation would follow the Strategic Plan, investment program and budget, annual submission of a progress report on Program implementation, and annual submission of a revised Strategic Plan, budget, investment program, work, training, and procurement plans (SAR, p. 43). The main security for IDA and other donors was in the annual review process at which time problems could be addressed and presumably solved. There were no special remedies included for poor performance. In the worst possible case the legal agreements fell back on the standard remedies: suspension and cancellation. As stated in the appraisal report, "If it should prove to be impossible to recommend a continuation of the sector-wide approach, as reflected in disagreements between IDA and the Government on the Strategic Plan, the investment program or the health budget, implementation would be halted and ultimately the credit would be cancelled" (SAR, p. 30).

SECTOR PROGRAM IMPLEMENTATION

Implementation experience:

(1) The reviews of past performance in April were typically less successful than the consultative prospective meetings in October/ November. One reason is that the progress reports prepared by the government were not particularly good, although they were comprehensive, and monitoring and evaluation capacity was weak. The prospective consultative meetings, by contrast, were held outside Lusaka and involved headquarters staff plus consultants from the various donor agencies. These meetings dealt in depth with issues concerning pharmaceuticals, reproductive health, financial framework, district capacity building, and standards for infrastructure. Concurrent working groups on the issues often were the same from year to year. The results of these deliberations often effected modifications in the Strategic Plan, or the joint donor/government statements.

(2) The annual meeting was effective, inter alia, because (a) it gave external agencies an opportunity to be involved and an opportunity to influence sector plans, and (b) it provided openness between government and donors. Other countries sent representatives to the annual meetings to observe the dialogue and deliberations. These representatives remarked on the openness of the dialogue, even on contentious issues.

(3) The Zambia program pioneered the use of "basket funding," or pooling of donor contributions into a common account. The idea of financing against the government budget started with the proposed DANIDA grant funds to districts. Although this idea did not materialize during the design stage, donors supported the concept during implementation. Donor funds were pooled for district grants and made use of common

accounting and reporting procedures developed with DANIDA assistance. Separate donor accounts were established at the center. They were released monthly and were commingled at the district level, i.e., donor origins could not be identified. The release of funds by the center was negotiated with all donors. Each donor had veto power.

(4) In practice, the Bank as a "donor of last resort" did not work particularly well because detailed budgets were never sufficiently developed against which expenditures could be justified. The Special Account (SA) became a slush fund. Whenever money was not available, the client went to the SA for funding, including staff allowances and housing for staff.

(5) During program development and implementation there have been four different ministers of health. The second minister tried to derail the reforms, but parliamentarians supported the health manifesto and brought him back into line. Broad approval was required to delink the health staff from the civil service (including defeating lawsuits), create the Central Board of Health, and make districts into autonomous boards. Thus, the reform had broad-based and high level support. Prior experiences with changes of leadership had not altered the directions of reform. However, all that changed in 1998. In 1998 a new minister of health was appointed. The new minister changed, not officially but in effect, priorities and placed emphasis on support for tertiary care institutions and centralization. This had the effect of reversing some reform strategies. The criticism was leveled that the reforms had not resulted in better service to beneficiaries. In addition, some serious issues arose about corruption in the pharmaceuticals stores. The new minister took an adversarial relationship with donors. The openness that had prevailed evaporated. The minister prevented an open

dialogue in the 1998 annual meeting. Implementation of the program came to a standstill. DANIDA suspended most of its program. Few funds have been disbursed from the credit in over one year. Several procurement applications have been rejected by the Bank.

(6) A Memorandum of Understanding was worked out among the donors, but was not signed because of the ensuing issues that developed in the subverting of the reforms.

(7) During implementation the Task Team Leader remained in Bank headquarters. The question arises whether problems would have been avoided by staff representation in the Resident Mission. On balance, this reportedly was not a hindrance. It made for about five missions per year, but perhaps also afforded the opportunity for the Bank to have a different perspective from other donor representatives who followed events daily from within the country.

(8) So far only one-third of the Credit proceeds have been disbursed after five years of implementation. The main reasons for the low disbursements were disagreements just before bulky disbursements on large contracts.

OUTCOMES SO FAR

Main achievements: Most of the progress achieved under the program was made in the first two years of approval of the IDA Credit. The areas of achievement were defined and actions were taken that had to be further developed, reinforced, and sustained in the remainder of the program implementation period.

(1) There has been a dramatic increase in the capacity of districts to plan and manage their affairs.

(2) In terms of reorganization and restructuring, the Central Board of Health was created as were autonomous hospitals and district boards.

(3) Health staff were started to be delinked from the civil service (this has now been halted).

(4) An essential package of care has been defined.

(5) The budget allocated to tertiary care has decreased in favor of budgets for the districts.

(6) In terms of actual impact the story is more mixed. Immunization coverage did increase and the demographic and health survey showed some improvements in terms of increased access to reproductive health and increased satisfaction with health services (in terms of cleaner facilities and more pleasant staff).

Main problems (or lack of achievements):

(1) Spending versus budget. The program has suffered from inappropriate spending within the health budget. The allocation to the social sectors has been maintained, in part through conditions imposed under adjustment credits. The Ministry of Health was getting the budget funds, but the funds were not getting distributed to intended beneficiaries. Pharmaceuticals were not financed (this was a major dispute in 1998). Care abroad (mainly for AIDS patients in South Africa) was amply financed, but district grants were underdisbursed (in 1998 only 60% of the budget was allocated). The causes for underspending in important categories was partly the result of inexperience with budgeting processes and underanticipation of needs. Another cause was lack of financial information. A third reason was overoptimism in ability to reallocate resources. The hospitals from which resources would be transferred to districts existed and could not be allowed to go bankrupt; they had to be sustained through the budget. The autonomous hospitals consumed 70% of the recurrent budget. Capacity building did not include strengthening the financial management of these entities.

(2) Pharmaceutical reform. This item was not on the agenda at the beginning of the reform program. The government did not want to discuss it. The first minister and the permanent secretary of health were fired over a drug scandal. This was a thorny issue because of the patterns of corruption involved in pharmaceuticals. (Astonishingly, the parastatal agency for drugs is now managed by an international arms dealing firm).

OBSERVATIONS AND POSSIBLE LESSONS

(1) The preparation process for the SIP took two years more than a traditional project would have taken. In part, this is because the Ministry of Health has taken the lead in shaping the implementation of health reforms. Ensuring that the Ministry remained the primary decision-maker often entailed moving at a slower pace than the project preparation team anticipated. The local sense of ownership and spirit of collaboration helped achievements in the early years of project execution.

(2) In hindsight, four years after the start of project implementation, it is clear that the directions for development of the sector were not fully explicit. There were no objectively verifiable indicators that could define adherence or deviation from the agreed plan. Too much was left to interpretation and opinion. The Bank did not agree with the Government and other donor partners on outcome indicators, indicative targets, and milestones for jointly monitoring the program. In retrospect, useful indicators would have been spending as a percentage of budgets on primary, secondary, and tertiary facilities; and availability of drugs. There should have been specific, clearly stated milestones, e.g., CBOH established with an acceptable memorandum of understanding between CBOH and the MOH; legislation

supporting decentralization passed, etc. It is therefore advisable first to get baseline data and agree on indicators and not to make commitments until there is explicit agreement on what constitutes progress.

(3) Thought should be given before commitments on how to resolve disputes – among the donors and between donors and the client. Does majority rule? Or is it weighted by how much each donor is contributing?

(4) Lack of linkages between performance and disbursements. Funds were not disbursed against performance and targets.

(5) Remedies: The legal language was not strong enough on agreement on the investment program. Funds were not released to districts and more funds were spent than planned on central MOH, CBOH and pharmaceuticals. The Bank did not have anything in the legal documents to deal with a situation in which distortions occurred in the program. There were no remedies short of suspension and cancellation. These are extreme measures that leave IDA isolated and without the means to continue the dialogue. The recommendation is: do not lend without recourse. Think of remedies from the first day of project development.

(6) A standard is needed to ensure that the Bank's role as donor of last resort works properly. The use of the Special Account became distorted in this case. A proper, comprehensive, and operable budget could have served as this standard, and should have been possible, but—as presented to the annual consultative meeting—was lacking in detail.

(7) The Zambia experiences show clearly how the SIP depended heavily on dialogue, which then broke down. There is no alternative if the dialogue breaks down.

(8) The case also shows the sensitivity of dealing with policy issues and the full sector program. This gets donors deeply involved in all aspects of the sector, which may be regarded by the client as interference and therefore cause resentment.

(9) One issue to be faced in a sector program is this: how do specific needs get covered when the attention is given to the overall program? For example, in health, how does one ensure that child health, AIDS, maternal health, and nutrition will get sufficient attention in the overall program? One method is to assign specific programs to particular donors and ensure that all programs are adequately covered. For IDA the dilemma is that it is perceived as not doing what it does not directly finance.

(10) The criticism of sector programs is that they focus more on process than on substance, impact, and outcomes. However, this misrepresents the issue. Process supports the changes required to achieve impact. The "production model" needs to be clearer in the health reforms.

(11) IDA involvement extends throughout the sector. Rather than only focusing on malaria, childhood diseases, the training of health cadres, facility renovation, drug selections, cost-recovery policies, or other "project" components, the Bank team is forced to be aware continually of any issues that might obstruct progress for the sector as a whole rather than the component being financed by the IDA Credit. This is more time-consuming and demands a greater familiarity with health sector issues than might otherwise be required. In a sector-wide approach considerable effort is needed to analyze the system and keep the knowledge of donors up to date. This requires continuing analysis, and reanalysis, such as expenditure reviews. It is costly. It cannot always be included in the loans/credits (it's not in the Government's interest sometimes to have these review of problems and progress). Supervision of a sector program takes at least 50% more budget than normal.

(12) The extent to which this approach depends upon effective donor coordination cannot be underestimated. Donors and government must remain in regular contact in order to recognize and respond to needs throughout the sector, for example, stepping in when critical sources of financing are delayed, or mobilizing a common response to policy decisions that might have an impact on the health sector. The interdependency inherent to the integrated sector approach has engendered and necessitated mutual trust and transparency. It also demands responsiveness, flexibility, and continuity on the part of Bank staff.

(13) Because inputs to the sector are better coordinated and because the government is encouraged to lead the process, the approach is expected to ensure better impact on health status and achieve more sustainable results. At the same time, it may mean that measurable outcomes are less readily obtained. It may be a trade-off between achieving short-term but unsustainable aims versus impact over a longer term that is sustainable. Reductions in morbidity/mortality of a specific disease could be more easily achieved under a disease-focused project, or progress in health personnel achieved if the project focused on training. It is more laborious to push the entire sector forward than to limit the scope to discrete projects that would produce more rapid measurable outcomes. Some consideration is now required as to how the Bank should measure success in such an integrated sector project.

BIBLIOGRAPHY

Joint Donor and Ministry of Health Statements. 1994, 1995, 1996, 1997.

Mahler, Halfdan, et al. 1997. "Comprehensive Review of the Zambian Health Reforms." Report of an independent review in September 1996. May 1997.

McLaughlin, Julie. 1997. "What Can We Learn from Implementation of a Sector-Wide Investment Approach to Lending?" Presentation at HNP Training Day for HD Resident Mission Staff. 19 March.

————. 1998. "Supervision Report: Zambia Health Mission". April 2.

Republic of Zambia Ministry of Health. 1998. "Memorandum of Understanding Between the Ministry of Health and Cooperating Partners in the Health Sector." July.

World Bank. No date. "Turning the Tables for Zambia's Health System." Handout in the "Investing in People" and "The World Bank in Action." Human Development Department.

World Bank. 1994. "Staff Appraisal Report, Zambia: Health Sector Support Project." Human Resources Division, Southern Africa Department, Report No. 13480-ZA. October 14, 1999.

TABLE 1
3239 – Zambia, Health Sector
Project Status Report Date: **6/30/99**

Region:	AFR	Country:	SENEGAL			Sector:	HH	Lending Instr:	SIL
Prg Obj Cat:	PA	EA Cat:	C	PTI?	Y	NGO?	Y	Resettlement?	N

LOAN INFORMATION

Agree Type	L/C/G No.	Orig Amt	Rev'd Amt	Currency Indicator	Prod Line	Signing Date	Effective Date	Suppl Prj ID
IDA	26600	38.70 (SDR)			PE	12/8/94	2/24/95	

Total Original Amount (SDR): 38.70   Total Revised Amount (SDR): 0.00

COFINANCING INFORMATION

Agency	Board Amount ($M)	Current Amount ($M)
DANIDA	20.00	20.00
DIGIS	60.80	0.00
NET	0.00	60.80
ODA	24.90	24.90
SIDA	21.20	21.20
UNICEF	14.00	14.00
Total	140.90	140.90

Guarantee Type: Guarantee Amount ($M):

This form is part of: **Supervision Mission**
Read together with:

( ) Aide-memoire	Mission End Date:	5/25/99	This Form PSR Date:	6/30/99
( ) BTO memo of:	Months since last mission:	6	Last Form PSR Date:	1/26/98
( ) Follow-up letter of: 6/15/99	Next mission planned:	11/1/99		

SUPERVISION EFFORT	Total Staff-Weeks	Total $000	Field Staff-Weeks	Field $000	As of 6/22/99
Current FY - Planned	30.50	110.59			
Current FY - Actual	26.63	92.25	0.00	0.00	
Board through preceding FY	236.05	664.70	50.15	152.73	
Total Actual	262.68	756.95	50.15	152.73	

UPI No.	Mission Member	Division	No. of Fld Days	Role or Specialization	Previous Mission
705	BERK	AFTH4	8.0	MISSION LEADER	Y
98421	FOLLMER	AFTH1	7.0	OPERATIONS	N
112460	KRISHNAKUMAR	AFTS1	5.0	PROCUREMENT	Y
175455	SIAMATOWE	AFMZM	10.0	SOCIAL SECTORS	Y
194952	MUMBA		10.0	PROCUREMENT	N
175456	MUSUNGWA	AFMZM	10.0	FINANCIAL MGMT	N

Ethiopia Education Case Study[1]
Education Sector Development Program (EDSP)

BACKGROUND

Ethiopia has the second largest population in Sub-Saharan Africa, but a per capita income of only about $110, one-fourth the average of the region. Nearly three decades of civil war and mismanagement through a centrally planned economy reduced the average per capita income in 1991 below that attained in 1960. The economy, however, embarked on rapid recovery and growth once the civil strife ended in 1991. Economic stabilization and reform programs contributed to an annual GDP growth of 5-8 percent in the first half of the 1990s.

As a result of previous neglect, Ethiopia's education sector is characterized at all levels by extremely low overall participation rates (30% at primary, 13% at secondary and less than 1% at tertiary levels). Its gross primary enrollment rate of 30 percent is one of the lowest in the world and less than half the average for Sub-Saharan Africa. Girls' participation rates are much lower than those of boys, especially in rural areas. In addition, there are severe urban-rural and regional differences in access to education (ranging from 7% in the Afar region to 87% in Addis Ababa). The quality of education is poor with inadequately trained and poorly motivated teachers and lack of instructional materials. The system is inefficient and one-third of students drop out of school in the first year. Physical facilities are in disrepair because of war damage and absence of preventive maintenance. Finally, the sector is seriously underfinanced.

To address the above issues the Government prepared a new Education and Training Policy and Strategy in 1994, which focused on restructuring, expanding, and improving the quality of the education system. This led to the creation of a 20-year Education Master Plan and an Education Sector Development Program (EDSP) covering the first five years of the long-term program. Donors were invited to participate in the final development and financing of the ESDP in late 1996. The Program was launched by the Government in 1997/8.

SECTOR PROGRAM DESIGN

Basic data: The EDSP is classified as a Sector Investment and Maintenance (SIM) in terms of the Bank's instruments. That is, it (a) is sector-wide in scope; (b) is based on an agreed program with all major donors; (c) contains a comprehensive expenditure plan in which the donors will finance a part; (d) is client-led; (e) incorporates efforts at using the and strengthening the client's procedures; and (f) includes harmonizing procedures; among the donors. The

---

[1] Based on two interviews with Mr. Arvil Van Adams, The Project Appraisal Document dated May 4, 1998, the Bank's "Quality at Entry Assessment" for CY 1998, and Martin, Oksanen, and Takala, "Preparation of the Education Sector Development Programme in Ethiopia," June 7, 1999.

Quality at Entry Assessment (QEA) states that "an APL would have been a preferable instrument. An APL would have forced the government, donors and the Bank to confront important issues of sequencing that are now dangerously implicit. It would have exerted some discipline on the donors. However, the Government refused to use an APL. The project now has implicit annual tranches, but no explicit triggers" (Section 1.5).

It took ten months for preparation of the ESDP, and from the March 1997 presentation of ESDP the program was delivered in just over one year, in May 1998. (See data sheet).

Rationale for the sector program: From the Government perspective, the problems in education were massive. Isolated projects were felt to provide an inadequate strategy for improving the situation. Specific projects in the past had tended to have limited impact (Martin, Oksanen, and Takala, p. 6). From the donor perspective, the sector program is a response to a Government-initiated sector program. One reason was therefore to support the Government-led initiatives. Another reason was the search for a more effective approach to external assistance. IDA, for example, had seven previous projects in the education sector and had relatively few accomplishments to show for it. Specific investment credits would continue to have limited impact, but a sector-wide approach was more likely to identify, address, and have success in solving the most critical issues for education as a whole. In addition, the sector-wide approach could avoid the "balkanization" or fragmentation of donor aid to the education sector. Moreover, harmonization of procedures could help ease the burden on Government of different procedures and PIUs insisted on by different donors.

Preconditions: First, the government had achieved a growth environment in the 1990s. It had the right macroeconomic policies, and GDP was growing an average of 7% annually, generating resources to support additional investment in the social sectors. Second, the Government had developed a credible sector program without donor intervention. Substantial Government ownership and commitment backed up the policy document. Third, there

was an adequate knowledge base for a sector-wide program, in part generated through an Ethiopian-executed PHRD grant.

Definition of the sector: ESDP is a sector-wide program that encompasses all education-related undertakings of the Government, both at the central and regional levels. (Program Appraisal Document [PAD], 14) The education "sector" covered by the ESDP is therefore comprehensive, including all levels and types of education. Specifically, the Program includes basic education, secondary education, technical and vocational education and training, teacher training, tertiary education (both formal and non-formal), special needs education, distance education, and institutional development. However, as reported in the QAE report, there is only a modest focus on secondary education, only a "studies position" on vocational training and little on tertiary education (section 1.4). All of the subsectors are within the purview of a single Ministry, the Ministry of Education. The unified management structure was a factor contributing to the success of program development (compared with, say, Zambia education, which involved four ministries).

Program leadership: A distinguishing characteristic is the strong leadership asserted by the Government. There was little donor involvement in the initial phase of the development of national policy and strategy. After the overall program was developed the Government invited donors to participate in financing it. This led to intensive collaboration between the Government and donors in detailed preparation of the program. In all aspects the Government was in the "driver's seat" for the program. Another characteristic was the continuity of staff on the central government side (although not in all the regions involved).

Donor coordination: The Government and other donors asked the Bank to lead the preparation of donor assistance to the Program and the missions to prepare the details of the program. Apart from formal meetings, the Task Team Leader spent enormous amounts of time with donors to ensure coordination of efforts. The need to collaborate with other donors takes some of the control out of the Bank's hands. For example, during program preparation a mission had to be delayed at the request of the EU because it could not field its team on time. The number of donors participating in ESDP preparation grew from 11 in the first mission to 15 by the final mission. A wide range of specialists were involved in the three preparation missions, and the number of each mission ranged from 19 on the first to 30 specialists on the third mission (Martin, et al., p. 7). One problem was that the technical specialists, often consultants, were not authorized to speak for the donor agency. This made it difficult to get official agency views on issues during the missions. One review of ESDP found that there was a "lack of forum for dialogue on policy and strategy development and management issues", and "by default, the team leader of the World Bank dominated the policy dialogue with the Government. This was the main single source of discontent from other donors" (Martin, et al., 2p4).

Program development: In parallel to ESDP the Government also undertook the preparation of the Health Sector Development Program (HSDP – see separate case). Many major meetings and supporting studies and design work were shared by ESDP and HSDP. ESDP preparation took place about six months ahead of HSDP, and lessons from the first could be taken into account in the second (e.g., size of missions, steps to follow, key documents to produce). Development of EDSP can be divided into three phases, each with the events listed below:[2]

Initiation Phase

(1) 1994: Education and Training Policy and Strategy prepared by Government; Education Master Plan (20 years) prepared by MOE; Short-Term Education Plan (5 years) with focus on primary education.

(2) 1995: Education Sector Investment Program prepared by Ethiopian consultant

(3) December 1996: Submission of ESDP to Consultative Group meeting in Addis Ababa. The government was somewhat resentful that donors wanted to question the program and carry on a dialogue about its content. After the meeting background papers were distributed to the donors for review in depth.

(4) March 1997: "Debre Zeit I" covering both education and health: Government-led workshop on social sector investment programs. The purpose was to get feedback from donors about the program and indicative budget support. It concluded with an overall positive assessment of the education program and a list of questions that needed to be investigated further, especially on capacity.

Preparation Phase

(1) May 1997: First joint donor technical assistance mission.

(2) Sept./Oct. 1997: Second joint donor technical assistance mission.

(3) January 1998: Study on "Implementing Sector Development Programs in Ethiopia".

(4) February 1998: Third joint donor technical assistance mission (i.e., appraisal).

Implementation Planning and Negotiations Phase

(1) April 1998: IDA follow up mission and negotiations in the field.[3]

---

[2] Martin, p. 4.

[3] IDA wanted wide participation by other donors in this mission, but the government refused to allow any donors to take part unless they would be bound by the resulting IDA agreement—which was not possible. An exception was made for the African Development Bank.

(2) May 1998: Study on "Harmonizing Requirements and Procedures Among Potential Funding Agencies Supporting Education and Health Sector Development Programmes in Ethiopia," focusing on monitoring, reporting, reviews, and evaluations. Board Presentation: May 26, 1998; and Credit Signing: June 12, 1998.

(3) September 1998: First complete version of Program Action Plan (PAP), a summary presentation of the ESDP; Study on "Financial Reporting System on the Use of Donor Funds."

(4) October 1998: Program Implementation Manual (PIM).

(5) November 1998: "Debre Zeit II" on both education and health. This was a wrap-up presentation of the final program to mobilize the support of other donors. However, war had started with Eritrea in May 1998, and further donor support was not forthcoming.

There was no overall plan or "grand design" for development of the Program from the stage of donor involvement. Nor was it overly prescriptive early in the process. An interactive, pragmatic approach was used. Key documents for agreements included the Program Action Plan (PAP), a five-year plan based on a summary of the various regional plans, and the Program Implementation Manual (PIM). The PIM spells out separately all the guidelines for ESDP implementation and includes practical guidelines for persons responsible for implementation. Topics covered include annual planning cycle; financial management; procurement management; construction management; and monitoring and evaluation.

The main substantive issue between IDA and the government had to do with vocational training. The overall program called for rapid vocationalization of schools. IDA raised questions about cost and linkages with the labor market. In the end the regions called for studies before adopting the central government's plan. The main procedural or administrative disagreement was over the structure of the central steering committee. The government wanted only three donors on the committee with a majority of government representatives. Furthermore, they wanted decisions by majority votes. This proposal left some donors out of the deliberations. The three donors could not commit the wider group of donors, and could not accept voting as a means of reaching decisions (compared with consensus). In the end it was agreed that the three donors on the steering committee would be advisors and not participate in decision-making on the project. A donors group was established to facilitate communication among the donors.

Level of sector analysis: As mentioned previously, the high level of sector analysis was one of the reasons for Bank acceptance of the sector-wide approach. Annual public expenditure reviews and a social sector expenditure review were available. In particular, the 1997 public expenditure review by the Bank established a medium-term expenditure framework. The bulk of the analysis that preceded the preparation of the ESDP was produced and facilitated by the PHRD project financed by a Japanese grant and executed by the Government. According to Martin (p. 5) the studies developed by the project generated primary data through household, institutional, and community surveys and combined this with secondary data from previous studies. The majority of the work was carried out by local staff and consultants. Nine separate studies were produced, including access to and supply of educational facilities; demand and supply of educational manpower; private and social returns to education; demographic analysis and population projections; household demand for schooling; the role of NGOs and private sector in service delivery; costs and financing of education; community consultation; and participation; and cost effectiveness of key educational inputs. In addition, the Bank's Task Team Leader spent considerable time with other donors to assemble analyses done by other agencies. In particular, USAID, the EU (on higher education), and SIDA (cost-effectiveness of different types of school construction) had significant studies and analyses that had not yet been widely disseminated.

Instruments for agreements: The main instruments for agreements were the documents produced by the Government (the Plan and Program), the agreements reached at a donor conference, and the aides-mémoire of the missions. In addition, the PAP and PIP provided a detailed basis for agreements on the program and its implementation. Late in the program development (at about the stage of effectiveness of the IDA Credit) some of the donors, e.g., SIDA, proposed the development of a Memorandum of Understanding (MOU). However, the Government was not receptive. The Government viewed this as just another hurdle and felt that existing documentation (the PAP and PIP) would suffice. There was no formal agreement between the Bank and other donors. In retrospect, the Task Team Leader felt that some kind of formal agreement would have been highly useful at the start of the process of detailed preparation, to define roles and responsibilities more clearly. This would have complemented the considerable goodwill that existed at that stage.

Institutional capacity: In the view of the Task Team Leader institutional capacity was not satisfactorily assessed during program preparation. In part this was because the government had difficulty throughout project preparation in accepting that it had weaknesses in institutional capacity, even under the decentralization program. The Office of the Prime Minister (OPM) did not recognize initially that it had a problem of institutional capacity to implement the program. The central Ministry of Education (MOE) had been a capable ministry in the past. However, it had been weakened by the overall Government program to decentralize public administration. Many experienced staff either were transferred to regions or left the MOE altogether rather than be reassigned. There was no clarity among remaining staff about the role of a central ministry in a decentralized setting. Several regions had reasonable administrative capacity, but at least three or four regions were almost hopelessly weak. No analysis seems to have been made about incentives of key actors in the implementation of the program (QEA, section 6.1). The problem was how to address the weak capacity. An external consultant was used on assessing institutional capacity, but without much success. During missions technical assistance was provided. For example, by examining the work to be done in transferring funds and implementing the program, officials came to see that the procedures, tasks, and capacity required had not been thought through sufficiently. The missions finally were able to achieve some modest success in introducing an institutional development component in the expenditure program covering support for information systems, human resource development, and hardware.

Stakeholder consultation: The process of program development was managed from the top down: first development of the central policy and framework, then preparation of regional plans. Regional plans were wholly developed by the various sections of regional education bureaus. However, few regions reported significant involvement of lower level stakeholders in the process, other than to provide data and information. A few regions held seminars or distributed draft plans down to the zonal level for comments. One city-region, Harari, had consultations with all its teachers, but in general information about the ESDP was not widely disseminated during the preparation process. Few persons outside of regional bureaus had more than a passing awareness of its existence. As stated in the QEA, "direct consultations with stakeholders are not evident to have been a part of the preparation of the program" (section 4.1). Still, the level of participation and decentralization of the planning process for ESDP in Ethiopia was far more widespread than in other comparable countries. Inclusion of some bottom-up processes would have been of great advantage, but would have taken more time and would have been more difficult to manage. Many regions are now taking steps to rectify the lack of dissemination, but it is difficult in larger regions (Martin, et al., p. 35).

THE SECTOR-WIDE PROGRAM

Objectives and content: The objectives of the first five-year phase of ESDP are to improve the overall educational attainment of the population while achieving greater social equity. The long-term objective is to achieve universal basic education by 2015. Targets for the first phase include increasing the primary enrollment ratio from 30% to 50% of the eligible population (from 3.1 million students to 7 million) with emphasis on rural areas; improving enrollment ratios for girls from 38% to 45%; improving efficiency by reducing dropout and repetition rates; improving quality and relevance by reducing the book to student ratio from 5:1 to 1:1 in core subjects; and improving financing by increasing public spending on education from 3.8% to 4.6% of GDP. The central Government has provided the overall framework, policy, and targets and each region has developed its own program reflecting local conditions and aspirations. The sum of the regional plans plus the central framework constitute the ESDP. In the primary education program, components include construction, renovation and upgrading of schools, curriculum reform, teacher training, and book provision. Secondary education includes expansion of facilities to reduce congestion, curriculum revision, upgrading of teachers, and provision of instructional materials and equipment. TVET includes employer and market surveys of needs. Teacher training includes upgrading and expansion of training capacity, introduction of distance teaching, and training of school managers. Tertiary education includes expansion in limited areas (education, engineering, health workers and public administration, and institutional analyses of cost-effectiveness. Institutional development includes support for planning, examinations, financial management, implementation, and monitoring and evaluation. Key policy reforms include extending primary education from 6 to 8 years, automatic promotion from grades 1-3, use of local languages in primary grades, establishment of a new career teaching structure, elimination of fees for grades 1-10, and the introduction of cost recovery in grades 11-12. ESDP also supports the government-wide program of decentralization in the education sector.

Organization and management: ESDP implementation is carried out through existing institutions, largely following existing Government procedures. However, the monitoring, coordination, and oversight of ESDP are carried out through bodies created for ESDP. These include a Central Joint Steering Committee and its Secretariat and their analogs in the regions, Regional Joint Steering Committees and corresponding secretariats (PAD, p. 14). The secretariats, in particular, are responsible for monitoring progress, managing information flows, and reporting and approving work plans. Regional Educational Bureaus have the responsibility of implementing about 87% of the program. The QEA report observed, "the program relies heavily on steering committees .... This may be the best that can be done in the situation, but steering committees ... cannot substitute for weak capacity" (section 6.2).

Modus operandi: The nature of donor support and supervision is different from project support that requires that details of the operation be spelled out and costs determined in advance. For program support, the key is agreement on program objectives and targets, and the process by which these objectives and targets will be achieved (p.14). The key process in the sector program is the annual review. The purpose is to (1) look backward and review progress against targets in the previous year and, based on this and any changes in circumstances, (2) look forward to agree on the expenditure and implementation plan for the coming year. The QEA report noted, "the creative design feature of an annual review process to agree on the program for the following year provides a mechanism for sequencing, prioritizing as well as protection for the Bank" (summary). Inputs required for the process are regional and national monitoring indicators, annual work programs and budgets, and implementation performance as reported in progress reports and validated by independent reviewers. Two joint supervision missions (jointly held by the Government and donors) also feed information into the annual review, as do the results of previously agreed ad hoc reports and analyses. Reports by implementing agencies include expenditure data for the previous six months, data on physical targets achieved, procurement status, performance coefficients (achievements divided by agreed targets), issues, and plans to resolve them.

The annual review process depends critically on the quality of information collected, transparency, and mutual trust. A key part of the annual review process is the monitoring indicators. A set of twenty basic indicators has been developed, including budget and expenditures, access, quality, efficiency, and equity (PAD, Annex 7).

Harmonization of donor procedures is also a key feature of implementation. As stated in the PAD (p.12), to lighten the administrative burden on the limited capacity of the Government at all levels, it was agreed to harmonize donor procedures for supervision, monitoring and evaluation, and reporting. These were not fully worked out prior to the start of the Program. Common procedures are not included for procurement, in part because work was being done on the topic separately. However, it did not materialize and now the government is saddled with different procurement systems with each donor.

Financing: The ESDP costs about $1.8 billion over five years with contingencies, of which the IDA Credit will finance $100 million, or 5.6%. Other donors agreed (as of 4/1/98) to finance another $180 million and the Government contribution is $1.3 billion, leaving a financing gap of about $220 million. The financing gap is to be filled by other donors, or by scaling back the program. The Bank agreed to be the "lender of last resort". According to Martin et al., this has helped smooth relations with other donors. However, in practice it has not worked because of delays in getting firm commitments from other donors. The program is not fully funded and the IDA Credit cannot completely fill the gap. The Bank's financial plan is flexible: (1) It can disburse against anything but civil service salaries; and (2) about two-thirds of the Credit proceeds are unallocated. Moreover, the pace of disbursements is dictated by the pace of procurement. The Bank can finance more than currently planned per year based on actual implementation performance. Part of the understanding between donors and Government is that all parties would operate only within the agreed program; no additional donors would be allowed to provide assistance outside the agreed framework.[4]

Financial flows and disbursements: Instead of creating new parallel systems for moving money under the project, the donors wanted to use Government channels as much as possible. Some donors argued for budgetary support, but many donors had concerns regarding whether funds would be used for their intended purposes through the Government's own financial systems. Most donors—including IDA —wanted to be able to account for the funds. This required the development of a system to tag the money and report on it for reimbursements. In the end multiple channels were agreed for disbursements. "Channel 1" is via the regular financial system of the government, from the central MOF to regional Bureaus of Finance and so on. Channel 1 is subdivided into "1a" (unearmarked budget support), and "1b" (earmarked funds). "Channel 2" is via the sector ministry, i.e., to the central MOE, then to regional education bureaus, etc. "Channel 3" is directly from the donor to the recipient agency, bypassing the Government budget system. Several donors (SIDA, Norway, Finland, and DFID) expressed interest in providing donor support. The condition is confidence in financial management, reports, and accounting. However, so far none has contributed to the project through this channel. The Bank is using "channel 1b," USAID and the Irish are continuing to disburse funds through Channel 3. The issue of financial management was identified as early as the second mission, but the Office of the Prime Minister refused to get the MOF and others involved. They simply wanted donors to use existing financial systems. An expenditure review helped produce an action plan for the improvement of financial management, but its implementation has

---

[4] A complication for IDA has arisen because the Bank's agriculture sector is proposing to add a unit for traditional medicine at the agricultural university and it not clear whether it can be added because it was not envisaged as part of the original program.

been slow. Some offices lack financial systems and others have heavy rates of vacant positions. It took over one year to get Government acceptance of the existence of a financial management issue. The Finance Ministry is expected to supervise the program at regional levels and seek replenishment of special accounts. The Government wanted to have a disbursement plan for $35 million in the first year. The Bank staff did not believe this was realistic, assuming a target of $15 million would be more appropriate. However the Bank agreed to give the Government the benefit of the doubt on implementation capacity and let the actual pace of implementation determine the level of disbursements.

Procurement: The Development Credit Agreement calls for normal procurement procedures, except that it is "liberal" about thresholds.

Risks and dangers: The sector program does carry different risks than a specific investment project. For one thing, the external donors have to be concerned with policy developments from top to bottom and from one side to the other in all regions. Under a sector program the donors try to use Government systems and procedures as much as possible. For financial management this entails a higher risk of misuse of funds than under carefully controlled project accounts. Another risk is the added complexity of dealing with the sector as a whole rather than a more limited enclave. One risk pertains to the harmonization of donor procedures on procurement and financial management reporting. The risk is that the harmonization may not be comprehensive, therefore placing considerable burden on the Government's limited capacity at all levels (PAD, p. 40). However, the project documentation does not address the very large risk of lack of capacity of the regional and central government. There is no discussion of possible exit strategies (QEA, section 8.2).

Conditionality: Formal targets for education financing include an increase from 3.8% of GDP to 4.6% and from 13% to 19% of government spending, plus subsector targets (from 46% at present to 65% of education spending for basic education). The main conditions relate to the implementation of the agreed annual work program, as evaluated and de-

cided at the annual reviews. Financing can be advanced based on good implementation performance. In effect, the project has "implicit annual tranches" (QEA, summary). A new credit is even possible when most of the current one is used. Disbursements can be advanced if the pace of work justifies it. On the other hand, the Bank has a "slow down" strategy based on the annual review of performance. For gross distortions or major failure to deliver, the Bank could decline to commit any funds for the following year. Also, the donors act in concert.

SECTOR PROGRAM IMPLEMENTATION

Implementation experience: The main event affecting implementation has been the outbreak of war between Ethiopia and Eritrea. This has caused several donors that had previously committed to help finance the sector program to pull back and delay disbursements. Specifically, the Nordic and U.K. assistance programs were considering channeling disbursements through "Channel 1a", but stepped back after the war started. In the first year of the conflict the Government maintained its level of expenditures on the social sector. However, recent information indicates that major cuts are expected in social spending in the second year. The Government did not indicate any plan to cut social spending during the annual review. However, shortly after the annual review, cuts of 30% in regional budgets were announced. These cuts will require backloading the disbursement schedule. In addition, a major increase has taken place in the financing of higher education, ostensibly to improve output capacity in public administration and teacher training. The extent of the increase was not made explicit during the annual review. These events have led to suspicions on the part of the donors that Government representatives were not transparent about real intentions during the review. Thus, transparency in the process of mutual and free exchange of information has not yet been achieved.

An instrument is needed to provide transparency, so everyone can see all documents and reports without harboring suspicions about ulterior motives. As a result of the war, efforts at the harmonization of procedures by donors have stopped. Experiences with the annual review cycle reveal weaknesses in reporting. In particular, the annual review did not receive complete information on expenditures over the previous six months. The monitoring and information systems need further work to function properly and indicate weaknesses in local capacity to produce the required reports. In contrast with a Government target of $35 million in disbursements for the first year, only $12 million was disbursed in the first year, including retroactive financing. The Government wanted to have an allocation of $55 million for implementation in the second year, but only got $35 million including a rollover of unspent funds from the first year. Despite all the preparations, the MOE had to request a supplemental budget to put IDA funds into the budget. This delayed implementation.

OUTCOMES SO FAR

Main achievements:

(1) One clear achievement has been the completion of the preparation process for the program. It is widely seen an as innovative program and many donors have indicated interest in participation.

(2) The number (16) of donor agencies agreeing on the content of the program.

(3) Government ownership of the program and the process and the consensus achieved— although it was from the top down from the PMO to Regions, Zones, Districts, and then to schools. The initial decision to embark on an ESDP was entirely on the Government's own initiative and was without pressure from the donor community (Martin, et al., p. 39).

(4) Perhaps the most significant achievement is the quality of regional plans developed throughout the country. A comparison of original with final drafts shows the sea

change in quality that occurred in the process. For example, regions introduced new strategies for non-formal education that were not originally envisaged. The capacity building achieved has been enormous in terms of regional planning.

(5) Even though more consultation could have been done, the extensive educational planning done in regions contributed greatly to broadening stakeholder participation, and understanding and ownership of the program.

(6) The dialogue has had an impact on policies and goals; for example, plans for vocationalization of secondary schools have been toned down as a result of discussions during which international experiences were explained.

POSSIBLE LESSONS AND FINAL OBSERVATIONS

ESDP is the first sector program in the education sector that is truly sector-wide in scope, and the first to commence from the Government's own policy framework (Martin, et al., p. 30).

(1) The main conditions contributing to the success of the program development and design were (a) the macro framework, which allowed the program to develop within a growth economy; (b) the extensive knowledge of the sector and its problems; and (c) the client taking leadership over the process. It may be unlikely that a sector program will succeed without these conditions.

(2) Considerable continuity of core personnel on both the Government and donor sides during program preparation was an important factor in its success. It allowed for the establishment of trust and good working relationships (Martin, et al., p. 46)

(3) A formal agreement would be highly useful at an early stage to define roles and re-

sponsibilities of both donors and the client. This should include the role of the lead donor, if any. This would have helped to avoid later disputes, e.g., level of donor representation in the steering committee. The amount of time required for consultation with donors cannot be overestimated. The partners need to be kept informed, their inputs need to be used and consensus needs to be achieved. The transaction costs are enormous.

(4) Since the sector program does not define all activities and have everything in place in advance, the mechanisms for dialogue and deciding these matters during implementation become of overriding importance.

(5) The process of getting mutual understanding of the issues and resolving them cannot be done overnight, as evidenced by the one year it took for the OPM to recognize there was a problem with financial management capacity.

(6) The ESDP had targets for the end of the program, but not interim targets against which to measure year-by-year progress.

(7) The Bank does not have to take the lead in sector program development on the side of donors. If it does, it should be prepared to spend extra resources to ensure that technical gaps are filled and ensure full consultations. In the case of Ethiopia education the preparation cost $600,000 compared with $350,000 on the average.

(8) The capacity of other donors to deal with technical issues and policy dialogue is often limited. One the one hand consultants are often used for technical work, but are not authorized to speak for the donor on policy issues. On the other hand, donor staff sometimes are ill-prepared for policy dialogue themselves.

(9) It was relatively simple to harmonize monitoring and progress reporting and move toward jointly conducted reviews and evaluations. It was much more difficult to deal

with differences on procurement and especially financial management. These were the most contentious areas throughout the preparation of ESDP. It would have been useful if the PIM, financial management study, and harmonization studies could have occurred earlier.

(10) It is advisable to see harmonization and integration with donor procedures as a medium-term process that will pass through a series of transitional forms (Martin, et al., p. 47)– such as the multiple ways financial flows were organized for ESDP.

(11) The financial contributions of the various donors differ considerably and this almost invariably means varying amounts of influence in policy discussions. In the ESDP some donors felt left out and that the policy dialogue process was dominated by the Bank. This suggests that a forum should be part of program design for specifically discussing education policy issues on the basis of relevant professional experience (Martin, et al., p. 44).

(12) Sector-wide coverage means that technical and vocational education training, and higher education are included, areas in which achieving consensus is much more demanding than basic education. It also means greater complexity and possibly greater difficulty in implementation. However, a sector-wide approach also allows the donors to check whether subsectoral allocations of the education budget are appropriate, e.g., for higher education. This would not be easy if only one subsector, e.g., basic education, were included.

(13) Throughout program development perceptions differed widely between the government and donors on the management capacity and institutional requirements of the implementing agencies, including financial management procedures of the government. These disagreements delayed analysis of critical issues, such as financial manage-

ment, and delayed agreements on the extent of technical assistance needed to build capacity. The gap in perceptions could have been narrowed or closed by starting with an analysis of institutional capacity (although admittedly it would have been difficult to persuade the government to accept and participate in such a study). The ESDP did not have everything ready and completed by the time of Credit approval. A sector program, unlike a project, simply will not have all the details completed by the time of commitment. The difference is that a sector program creates a framework for the dialogue on issues. The question is: what is the critical threshold for going ahead with the program? In the case of the ESDP the IDA team was satisfied that it had 80% of what it wanted. It would take another five years to get the rest. The process for dialogue allows for the lose ends to be tied during implementation.

(14) The QEA pointed out that the government's development of the strategy before donor involvement means strong borrower commitment. However, "ultimately the Bank has to weigh client responsiveness against a very complex (and inadequately sequenced) strategy in a context of weak capacity and with multiple donors. … The prospects for success of the ESDP depend on the Bank and Borrower's ability to prioritize, focus and sequence the effort into more manageable elements" (summary). The annual review process provides a mechanism for doing this.

BIBLIOGRAPHY

Martin, John, and Riitta Oksanen, and Tuomas Takala.1999. "Preparation of the Education Sector Development Programme in Ethiopia: Reflections by Participants." Cambridge Education Consultants, UK and FTP International, Finland. Final Report, 7 June 1999.

World Bank. 1998. "Program Appraisal Document on a Proposed International Development Association Credit in the Amount of US$100 Million Equivalent to the Federal Democratic Republic of Ethiopia for the Education Sector Development Program." Human Development IV and Country Department 6, Africa Region, Report No. 17739-ET, May 4, 1998.

World Bank. 1999. "Quality at Entry Assessment: Guidance Questionnaire" as part of the Quality At Entry Report for CY 1998, on the Ethiopia Education Sector Development Program. (Communicated by Dora Aku Adoteye to Prem Garg, EM 10/8/99.)

TABLE 1
732 – Ethiopia, Education Sect. Inves
Project Status Report Date: **2/26/99**

Region:	AFR	Country:	ETHIOPIA			Sector:	EP	Lending Instr:	SIM
Prg Obj Cat:	PA	EA Cat:	C	PTI?	Y	NGO?	N	Resettlement?	N

LOAN INFORMATION

Agree Type	L/C/G No.	Orig Amt	Rev'd Amt	Currency Indicator	Prod Line	Signing Date	Effective Date	Suppl Prj ID
IDA	30770	74.30 (SDR)			PE	6/4/98	12/2/98	

Total Original Amount (SDR):	74.30	Total Revised Amount (SDR):	0.00

COFINANCING INFORMATION

Agency	Board Amount ($M)	Current Amount ($M)
Total	0.00	0.00

Guarantee Type:	Guarantee Amount ($M):

This form is part of: **Initial Summary**
Read together with:

( ) Aide-memoire	Mission End Date:		This Form PSR Date:	2/26/99
( ) BTO memo of:	Months since last mission:		Last Form PSR Date:	
( ) Follow-up letter of:	Next mission planned:	7/1/98		

SUPERVISION EFFORT	Total Staff-Weeks	Total $000	Field Staff-Weeks	Field $000	As of 2/26/99
Current FY - Planned	56.70	195.73			
Current FY - Actual	14.35	63.58	0.00	0.00	
Board through preceding FY	0.00	0.00	0.00	0.00	
Total Actual	14.35	63.58	0.00	0.00	

UPI No.	Mission Member	Division	No. of Fld Days	Role or Specialization	Previous Mission

The Gambia Education Case Study[1]
First Phase of the Third Education Sector Program

ACRONYMS

DFID	Department for International Development
DOF	Department of Finance
DoSE	Department of State for Education
EU	European Union
PAD	Project Appraisal Document
SIP	Sector Investment Program
SWAP	Sector-wide approach

BACKGROUND

The Government developed a 15-year strategy to improve education in the late 1980s, the *Sector Policy Framework (1988-2003)*. The priorities were to (1) increase the gross enrollment ration in grades 1-6 to 75% and the transition rate from grades 6-7 to 60%; (2) lower the school entry age from 8 to 7; (3) develop a broad-based curriculum for basic education (grades 1-9); (4) improve the quality of learning in the basic cycle by upgrading all unqualified teachers, increasing expenditures on learning materials; (5) increase access to post-secondary vocational training and coordinate its provision better; and (6) increase opportunities for out-of-school youth,

school leavers, and adults. During the 1990s the Government increased public expenditures on education at 10% annually in real terms. This resulted in an increase in spending on education from 15%-21% of total government expenditure and from 2.6% - 4.3% as a share of GDP. The proportion devoted to primary education also increased from 38% to 45% of the education budget. Gross enrollments in grades reached 70% in grades 1-6 and the transition rate from grade 6 to 7 increased from 35% to 70%.

Development of the education system is affected by several exogenous factors, including high population growth, which makes it difficult to keep up with service provision, limited public revenue and high debt service (30% of recurrent expenditure), which limits public resources available for education, and high levels of poverty in rural areas which affects the demand for education. The main issues internal to the education system are: (a) the need to expand enrollments by 8% per year to reach a 90% gross enrollment in the nine-year basic education by 2005, including accommodating an additional 175,000 students, and overcoming barriers to attendance particularly among girls and the poor; (b) unclear effectiveness of education in terms of learning achievements of students; (c) questionable equity and efficiency of public financing of education, in

---

[1] This case is based on interviews with Ms. Rosemary Bellew, Task Team Leader, and the Project Appraisal Document, "Third Education Sector Project In Support of the First Phase of the Third Education Sector Program," August 7, 1998, Report No. 17903-GM.

terms of available spending for poor students, insufficient expenditures on improving learning conditions, undersized classes, and high expenditures on untargeted subsidies (PAD, pp. 5-6).

The second half of the 15-year policy period maintains the same priorities and builds on these accomplishments while pushing for a target of 90% of the school age population enrolled in the 9-year basic cycle by 2005. It also pursues interventions to improve equity, effectiveness, efficiency, and building sector management capacity as well as issues in higher education and sector financing. The Government's objectives and strategies for addressing the issues have been refined and elaborated in the following documents: *Revised Education Policy, 1988-2003*, which updates the original policy, the draft *Master Plan and Investment Program, 1998-2005*, which describes priority programs, resource requirements, implementation responsibilities and schedules, and the *Public Expenditure Review, 1998*, which lays out policy decisions regarding intra-sectoral financing (PAD, p. 8).

SWAP DESIGN

Rationale for a sector-wide approach: The reasons for adopting a sector-wide approach are rooted in the shortcomings of previous project lending. The PAD states that a project approach to the development of the sector led to insufficient ownership and integration of project activities into the DoSE's work program (p.17). In addition, a sector-wide approach is adopted because of the negative effects of focusing in the past on only one subsector (basic education) through separate small projects. Projects limited to basic education had two negative effects: (a) donor concentration of funds in one subsector meant that public development expenditure, being fungible, was directed at other levels of education; and (b) development of the whole sector was not monitored. Moreover, the pad points out that all levels of education are linked to each other pedagogically and all derive resources from the same budget. Development of one subsector at the expense of others can distort

the necessary subsectoral linkages and result in a poor mix of products (PAD, p. 15). The sector-wide approach permitted the bank to seek policy objectives in higher education that otherwise would have been off-limits in a sub-sector approach. Specifically, the Bank has been discussing policies on reducing subsidies and introducing cost recovery in post-secondary education. (PAD, p. 12). Finally, it was felt that a sector-wide approach would help overcome some of the other problems associated with past projects, namely: overall weak management, planning, monitoring, and evaluation combined with a lack of consultation with stakeholders that resulted in poorly mapped-out strategies and implementation plans, lack of clearly defined responsibilities, the questioning of some strategies, and incomplete implementation or a reversal of the policy decision. The sector-wide approach involved extensive stakeholder consultations, preparation of annual implementation plans and annual review of program implementation, and strengthened administrative capacity, such as for monitoring and evaluation (PAD, pp. 17-18).

Lending instrument: The program lent itself to an Adaptable Program Lending (APL) instrument, as a transition toward a Sector Investment Program (SIP). (1) As noted above, the program is sector-wide in scope. (2) It includes well-defined overall objectives, strategies, and programs. Several of these need further conceptual work, planning, and budgeting (particularly vocational training and higher education), and thus are deferred to a second phase. (3) Medium- and long-term public expenditure plans have been estimated taking into account the macro-economic framework. (4) Local client is in charge of the process. However, the following elements of a SIP were not fully present: (a) all main donors agree to the program and commit to finance a share of the costs; (b) harmonization of donor requirements and procedures; and (c) reliance on normal government institutions and procedures for such things as procurement and financial management. Specifically, the DoSE did not have the initiative to effect strong coordination of donors. Only a limited number of multilateral and bilateral partners were interested in supporting the sector, and the volume and timing of their support was uncertain. Existing government capacity for management, monitoring and evaluation capacity was considered relatively weak (PAD, p. 15). Measures are included in the first phase to build necessary capacity as the program progresses.

Preconditions: Several factors were important in the decision to develop a sector-wide program approach. First, the Government had achieved a reasonable level of macroeconomic stability that provided a context for medium term planning of expenditures. Second, the Government had developed a 15-year policy framework which was decent and well done. The overall plan both demonstrated the Government's commitment to the process and the basic competence to develop reasonable strategies and programs. The Government was about halfway through the implementation of the plan. Third, a social sector expenditure review had helped build some capacity locally on how to do expenditure analysis. This analysis revealed the lack of congruence between policies and expenditures. Fourth, the Bank had a long history of dialogue with the Government through its previous two projects in education, the last of which allowed the start of discussion on policies. Fifth, the Bank had a consistent team, with whom the Gambian officials had gotten comfortable with. The level of confidence and trust allowed the Bank to push on issues, both with the DoSE and the Finance Ministry.

Definition of the sector: The "sector" includes all education and training at all levels. Specifically the sector is defined to include basic education, early childhood development, secondary education, vocational education and training, university education, adult education, and management and administration. All these subsectors are under the purview of one Ministry, the Department of State for Education (DoSE).

Program leadership: Leadership, ownership, and commitment have been demonstrated in a variety of ways by different Government entities. (a) The Ministry of Finance led the overall expenditure review. The Bank and DoSE worked together to analyze expenditures and the MOF participated in discussions of strategy development. The DoSE took the driver's seat in the preparation of the strategy and plans. The revised policy framework, investment program, and implementation plan, supported by a public expenditure review, were prepared by the DoSE with little or no input from technical assistance. Initially, the DoSE was not well organized to carry out this work, but the Permanent Secretary appointed a highly competent person to take charge of the work and the senior management team—which existed previously but was not functioning—provided the linkage between the overall picture and specific components throughout the process of development. (b) To ensure a high level commitment, the revised policy framework and investment program were discussed with and approved by the National Assembly. (c) In addition, a cabinet paper has been prepared and discussed to ensure appropriate support for budgetary allocations (PAD, p. 18). In the end it was clear to all that the Gambian side had prepared the strategy, program, and plans, not external donors.

Donor coordination: This was a relatively unique situation for Sub-Saharan Africa. About ten donors[2] have been active in The Gambia or have plans for projects in the near future. However, for various reasons, including the political situation, not a lot of donors were clamoring to provide support to the overall program. Initially the Bank did all the donor coordination and worked closely with other agencies such as UNDP, UNICEF, ADB, and WFP. However, by the time of appraisal the DoSE had appointed a donor coordinator. During appraisal, the DoSE convened partners to discuss modalities for partner coordination. The DoSE decided that donor coordination would be the responsibility of a team comprised of the DoSE coordinator, a representative of the external financing partners, the NGO community, the Department of Finance, and the Office of

---

[2] ADB, DANIDA, DFID, EDF, IDB, OPEC, UNDP, UNICEF, WFP, and the World Bank.

the President. UNICEF was appointed to represent the donor community. No major disagreements occurred among the donors. The DfiD and EU initially were reluctant to participate for political reasons, but eventually agreed to participate on a small scale.

Program development: Preparation of the Program took place piece by piece. The Bank helped Gambian officials analyze and work through various issues. It was important that Bank staff were available frequently for assistance and as a sounding board. This involved frequent missions. The key steps were as follows: (1) In 1995 the DoSE undertook its own review of progress under the 15-year program to determine what worked, what did not, and issues that needed to be addressed. Discussions were held in regional districts and culminated in a national conference at which conclusions were drawn. (2) Several specific evaluations were undertaken of such topics as double shift teaching and the book system. (3) The work on the public expenditure review with the Bank helped identify some additional issues for study. (4) As the results came in from the above specific studies, the DoSE prepared the Revised Policy Framework. (5) In parallel, the DoSE started working on the program document, with assistance from the Bank on a step-by-step basis, i.e., analysis of causes of major problems, examination of options in terms of cost and possible impact. This step included pre-appraisal. (6) Appraisal focused on finalizing costs, reaching decisions on cost recovery and teacher training and preparation of the implementation schedule. In this process the Government took several basic decisions on thorny issues, including: cutting back the number of unqualified teachers, reducing subsidies for school bus service, cutting subsidies to post-secondary students, attaching the issue of the high cost of examinations and scaling back and targeting the school lunch program.

Level of sector analysis: The three key statements of objectives and strategy for the program[3] identify key issues and select policies, programs, and resource requirements. The analyses underpinning the identification of issues and choice of strategies and objectives are contained in household surveys, preparation studies, and other sector work carried out during implementation over the past ten years during the implementation of the first half of the investment program (PAD, p. 8). Specific studies were generated during program preparation on subsidies to private schools, school feeding, overstaffing, inefficiency of the Gambia College and heavy subsidies to students in tertiary education. The DoSE had developed data collection that permitted time-series information to underpin the analysis.

Institutional capacity: One of the unique characteristics of the Gambia education APL is the systematic evaluation that was done of institutional capacity. This followed a methodology that analyzed all the proposed activities in the Program in terms of five criteria: whether (a) the functions and activities have an appropriate organizational home; (b) the level of leadership and management is effective; (c) sufficient operating funds are available for the implementation of assigned activities; (d) the unit has the right number of people with the right mix of skills—based on a workload analysis; and (e) key work practices are efficient and effective. This assessment identified several capacity gaps. For example, the analysis found that curriculum development and in-service teacher training had improper management responsibility outside the MoSE. Another example, in terms of work practices, was the weak coordination among units in the DoSE. The next step was to consider alternatives to fill the capacity gap through (i) changed practices and procedures, (ii) spreading activities over a longer time —including the introduction of a two-phase approach and postponement of some activities to the second phase; (iii) reallocating financial and human resources; and (iv) reducing the scope of the devel-

---

[3] *Revised Education Policy, 1988-2003*; the draft *Master Plan and Investment Program, 1998-2005*; and the *Public Expenditure Review, 1998.*

opment objectives. In the end the Gambia educa-tion APL included a detailed analysis of all major institutional components involved in the overall pro-gram and detailed capacity building measures (PAD, E4 and Annex 5).

Stakeholder consultation: Considerable stake-holder consultation took place in the design of the Program. The process began in 1996 with regional focus groups, followed by a national conference. Drafts of the program documents were discussed with NGOs, the teachers' union, representatives of the madrashas, the cabinet, the National Assembly and key development partners (PAD, p. 8).

THE PROGRAM

Objectives, strategy, and content: The IDA Credit sup-ports the implementation of the second half of the Government's long-term education program, i.e., over the period 1998 and 2006. The IDA assistance is divided into two four-year phases. The Program seeks to achieve a gross enrollment ratio of 90% in nine years of basic education; an increase of girls' enrollment and retention in the first twelve grades; improvements in the quality of basic education as measured by achievements on standardized tests; de-velopment of a program for early childhood devel-opment; increasing the gross enrollment ratio in secondary education from 16-25% along with im-provements and reductions in unit costs; improving the relevance of technical and vocational education through market surveys, policy development; up-grading of selected post-secondary programs to de-gree level in fields in demand; development of adult education programs and building sector management through improved organization of the DoSE, strengthened leadership, adjusting key work prac-tices, raising staff skills, and better mobilization and allocation of funds. These objectives entail new con-struction and rehabilitation of facilities, expansion of double-shift and multi-grade teaching, improve-ment in the supply and deployment of teachers, in-centives and subsidies for the poor and girls, an increase in the proportion of female teachers, wider distribution of textbooks and teaching materials, and the development of a national assessment system and improvements in examinations.

Organization: The DoSE is responsible for the implementation of the overall program and the IDA Credit. It does so through an interagency Project Co-ordinating committee, which it chairs, and a Coor-dination committee made up of representatives of the various units within DoSE. A Project Coordina-tion Unit (PCU) in the DoSE communicates with donors, coordinates program inputs, oversees pro-curement, provides financial management of IDA funds, and submits reports to all donors. The PCU previously existed as a project implementation unit. It was integrated into the MoSE and its terms of ref-erence were changed to purge all functions pertain-ing to implementation. Most[4] implementation functions were "mainstreamed" to line agencies.

Modus operandi: Partner coordination meetings take place at four-month intervals. The DoSE orga-nizes an annual meeting of all participating part-ners and the Department of State for Finance in May/ June each year. The purpose is to review (a) the progress in the implementation of the program, in-cluding staffing and expenditures; (b) the program of activities for the following school year; and (c) the draft development and recurrent budget. Changes can be made in the program and budgets revised based on actual experience and current circum-stances. The monitoring and evaluation arrange-ments are extremely important for the annual meetings. A set of quantitative monitoring indica-tors (Annex 4 of the PAD) has been developed per-taining to access, internal efficiency, budgets, resource utilization and expenditure, and availability and use

[4] The management of school construction remains in the PCU for the time being because the DoSE does not have an infrastructure unit in which this function could be mainstreamed.

of instructional materials. The DoSE updates these indicators annually, and prepares a comprehensive report on implementation performance before the annual meeting. A Management Information System is being developed, to be operational by 2001/2 to assist with this work. The Program does not yet entail much in the way of harmonization of procedures among the various donors, but supervision missions would be conducted jointly among the donors.

Financing, flow of funds, and disbursements: The overall program fits within an agreed expenditure framework. IDA financing is being provided in two phases: $20 million for phase I (1998-2003) and $20 million for phase II (2003-2007). The total cost of phase I is $51.3 million, of which the government would finance 18%, the Bank 39% and other donors 43%. The bulk of the Bank's funds in the first phase (64%) would be allocated to basic education, with 5% for secondary education, 3% for university education, 1% for adult education, and 9% for sector management. In effect, the Bank's financing is fixed for the first two years of implementation – similar to a Specific Investment Credit—but may be shifted during annual reviews based on performance, immediate priorities, and the interests of other donors (i.e., if other donors wish to finance certain aspects of the program, IDA funds can be shifted to other priorities). In addition, 16% of the Credit proceeds are unallocated for the second two years of the first phase and will be allocated during annual reviews (PAD, p. 15.) The support by other donor partners was not set at the time of the Credit commitment. IDA Credit funds are administered as in traditional projects, using statements of expenditures for relatively small purchases and a special account. Procurement also follows standard IDA practices for specific investment projects.

Risks and dangers: No special risks are identified in the PAD with regard to the sector-wide approach. Sustainability of project benefits depends, in part, on the avoidance of parallel programs supported by off-budget expenditures (PAD, p. 22) and continued stakeholder consultation and feedback. Implementation of the management capacity building component is seen as an antidote to the danger of weak implementation capacity of the DoSE.

Conditionality: Apart from routine conditions related to accounting procedures, appointment of auditors, and signature of contracts with supplier organizations, the main conditions under the APL relate to triggers for the second phase of the program. These include:

The triggers mix substance and process, of highly specific and unidentified targets. The key process of annual review and planning meetings is stressed, as is the use of common indicators. Annual agreements on budgetary allocations are also stressed, and the specific targets are included in the master budgetary plan and policy document that is cross-referenced in the Credit Agreement. No conditions were included on vocational training or higher education.[5] Apart from the standard suspension and cancellation clauses, the Bank's main leverage and "remedy" is in (a) varying the level of funding for the next year agreed on during each annual review, and (b) whether to proceed with financing the second phase of the APL.

SWAP IMPLEMENTATION

Implementation experience: Supervision of the Credit has been passed on the Bank's side from headquarters to the Bank's resident mission in Senegal—in

---

[5] On higher education, the Bank team felt that the risk for creation of a big university, as pushed for by the Presidency, was not great: After much discussion a phased plan had been agreed on to create a university in phases, starting with only two or three areas of demonstrated demand. Besides, there were no funds to support a major expansion. On vocational training the Government was not proposing to invest until studies were completed on better utilization of existing capacity and the roles of the public and private sectors were clearly delineated.

TABLE 1

Trigger	Indicator
Donor coordination is effective	❖ Annual review meetings organized and held by DoSE
	❖ Common monitoring indicators adopted and used
Access to basic education is increased	❖ Three-fourths of IDA-financed classroom construction is completed
Textbook recycling and rental systems are functioning	❖ All students in grades 1-6 have a set of textbooks to use free of charge
	❖ Rental recovery rates not less than 85% for grades 7-9
Teacher training capacity increases	❖ Gambia College takes in 300 PTC and 150 HTC teachers annually
Sufficient recurrent budget is allocated to education	❖ Annual budgetary allocations materialize as agreed

Source: PAD, p.4.

part to reduce the administrative costs of supervision and facilitate closer monitoring of implementation. Some problems were experienced during the startup phase. The Minister and Permanent Secretary (PS) changed. The PS in particular was not up to the job. This slowed progress several months, even though the technical people on the Government side were the same. However, in December 1998 a new PS was appointed who previously had led the technical work on the project. Since then things have started to move. The first annual review was scheduled for the fall of 1999.

Main achievements so far: It is very early in the implementation of the program, but some accomplishments can be noted for the design and preparation stages:

(1) Several significant policy decisions were taken on issues that had been hanging around for a long time, including unqualified teachers, subsidies of school bussing, school meals and subventions for students in higher education.

(2) DoSE staff got together behind the program, based on their participation in its development and understanding of its contents. This cohesion contrasts with the prevailing fragmentation within the department previously.

(3) Donors also reached common agreement on the program, which bodes well for avoiding the fragmentation of the past.

(4) Ownership: The DoSE made sure that everyone knew it was their program, not that of donor agencies. In the past projects were referred to by the donor, e.g., an ADB project or an IDA project, not a client-owned project. This program was different – it was owned by the people who prepared it. This can be seen by the enthusiasm of the staff to be engaged in the program development and implementation.

(5) Integration: Transforming the project implementation unit into a coordinating and support agency, integrating it within the DoSE and mainstreaming implementation functions with line agencies.

(6) Significant capacity building occurred. Staff were trained and became capable on modeling through the public expenditure review. Staff were trained in workload analysis and analysis of gaps in institutional capacity. Study tours for staff were undertaken on school effectiveness issues, economic analy-

sis, educational technology, and issues in higher education.[6] An expenditure model was developed that follows the normal budget categories and can be used for future projections and provide rolling guidance on whether budgets are on track.

(7) One major achievement is the systematic analysis of institutional capacity that took place during pre-appraisal and appraisal and successfully identified the important gaps in structures, procedures and resource allocations for the implementation of the program.

Main problems: The main problem in the design stage had to do with the capacity of local staff and institutions to prepare the program. It was difficult or impossible to find good economists or local architects. The organizational culture militated against staff working together and communication systems had to be designed to keep information flowing to all parties.

OBSERVATIONS AND POSSIBLE LESSONS

(1) The importance of thorough institutional analysis as a means to identify areas in need of strengthening, and thereby enhancing, the chances for successful implementation of the program.

(2) The use of a computerized model can serve a dual purpose: in addition to the evaluation of strategic alternatives it can also help track the key monitoring indicators during implementation.

(3) The startup experience for the Gambia Program demonstrates the importance of continuity of staff on the Borrower side. The situation was saved, in part, owing to the widespread consultation of stakeholders in the design phase, and the wide participation of technical specialists within the DoSE.

(4) The importance of frequent contact between government officials and specialists from the Bank (as opposed to periodic missions).

(5) The Government also emphasized the importance of good technical skills on the mission and proper timing of the visits.

(6) Several Gambian officials observed that it would have been helpful to have had the preparation strategy mapped out at the start. In that way everyone could see where it was headed and what it involved. However, if the process had been mapped out from the start it may have appeared overwhelming and new tasks might not have been as easily accommodated.

---

[6] The study tours travelled to (a) Colombia and Chile for "escuela nueva" (multi-grade teaching, modular curricula, etc), student assessment systems, decentralization, voucher schemes; (b) Washington for a range of topics—logical framework, higher education, education technology, economic analysis, and public expenditure reviews; (c) Addis Ababa for distance education for teacher training courses; (d) Mauritania for community-managed school construction programs; (e) to Senegal for adult literacy programs provided by non-government providers, and student assessment; (f) Ireland for higher education.

TABLE 2
35643 – The Gambia, Third Education
Project Status Report Date: **6/12/99**

Region:	AFR	Country:	GAMBIA			Sector:	EY	Lending Instr:	APL
Prg Obj Cat:	PA	EA Cat:	C	PTI?	Y	NGO?	N	Resettlement?	N

LOAN INFORMATION

Agree Type	L/C/G No.	Orig Amt	Rev'd Amt	Currency Indicator	Prod Line	Signing Date	Effective Date	Suppl Prj ID
IDA	31280	15.10 (SDR)			PE	9/22/98	3/22/99	

Total Original Amount (SDR):	15.10	Total Revised Amount (SDR):	0.00

COFINANCING INFORMATION

Agency		Board Amount ($M)	Current Amount ($M)
	Total	0.00	0.00

Guarantee Type:		Guarantee Amount ($M):	

This form is part of: **Supervision Mission**
Read together with:

( ) Aide-memoire	Mission End Date:	5/16/99	This Form PSR Date:	6/12/99
( ) BTO memo of:	Months since last mission:		Last Form PSR Date:	5/4/99
( ) Follow-up letter of: 5/25/99	Next mission planned:	10/1/99		

SUPERVISION EFFORT	Total Staff-Weeks	Total $000	Field Staff-Weeks	Field $000	As of 6/12/99
Current FY - Planned	0.00	0.00			
Current FY - Actual	18.15	69.22	1.00	9.09	
Board through preceding FY	0.00	0.00	0.00	0.00	
Total Actual	18.15	69.22	1.00	9.09	

UPI No.	Mission Member	Division	No. of Fld Days	Role or Specialization	Previous Mission
18303	DIAWARA	AFMSN	10.0	SR. OPS. OFFICER	Y
22339	DIOP	AFTH3	6.0	EDUCATION SPEC.	N
89807	TOURE	AFMSN	3.0	PROCUREMENT SPEC.	N
52149	HAGO	AFTH2	14.0	EDUCATION SPEC.	N
184936	NDIAYE	AFMSN	3.0	FINANCIAL MGMT SEP.	N

Mozambique Education Case Study[1]
Education Sector Strategic Program (ESSP)

The impetus for preparing the SWAP was Government's desire to develop a coherent strategic framework and a coordinated structure for the reconstruction and further development of the sector following the civil war. The response to dealing with the devastation of physical assets and social disruption that had taken place during the war was ad hoc and piecemeal. Bilateral and multilateral agencies and NGOs responded by providing assistance directly to beneficiaries using their own unique solutions to problems. As the country settled after the war it was difficult to systematically link the government's sector and fiscal policies with the efforts of external donors because of lack of information and sometimes conflict in approaches.

The World Conference on Education for All (Jomtien) was an added impetus for the Government of Mozambique (GOM) to develop a number of subsector master plans.

GOM's concern with increased coordination coincided with disenchantment on the part of the donors about the increasing ineffectiveness of their assistance. As the volume of aid increased, it became difficult for the country to absorb assistance without a coherent strategic framework, and GOM's capacity to coordinate assistance from a multiplicity of sources was stretched. Agreement on a SWAP approach was therefore mutual.

Low quality of primary and secondary education: Low quality constrains the efficiency of the system and limits the number of well-qualified students graduating from each level. Only 54% and 37% of students pass the grade 5 and grade 7 examinations, respectively. Although improving, internal inefficiency is apparent in high repetition and dropout rates and low completion rates. Barely 25% of students who enter the first grade successfully complete the five grades of lower primary. Only 7% of pupils enrolling in grade 1 complete grade 5 without repeating. Even those students who manage to stay in school are not learning enough because inadequate, bare facilities do not create a classroom environment conducive to learning, and multiple shifts reduce learning time. The number of learning hours per pupil per year has decreased by about 30% (from 850 to 595 hours) in lower primary education in recent years in some schools. This is lower than the modest 780 hours recommended by UNESCO.

SITUATION PRIOR TO ESSP

Prior to ESSP external assistance to MOE was provided under more than 150 different projects and subprojects, by more than 16 countries, numerous

---

[1] This case was drafted by the ESSP Program Secretariat with inputs from the Minister of Education, Hon. Minister Nhavoto, as supplemented by an interview with the Task Team Leader, Mr. Donald Hamilton and Operation Officer, Mr. Soren Nellemann, plus information from the Project Appraisal Document (PAD), January 22, 1999.

UN agencies,[3] multilateral financing institutions,[2] international bodies[4] and a large number of local and international NGOs operating throughout the country. In addition to the inability of the government to monitor the large number of projects, there were serious inequities in resource allocation to schools, districts, and provinces, and more important, resources were often not geared toward urgent priorities. In addition, the numerous PIUs and external agencies carried out similar exercises such as audits, supervision, etc., drawing heavily on the limited Government capacity, thereby reducing the Government's resources to undertake their administrative function. This was compounded by the use of different procedures and financial management systems by donors in parallel operations.

DESIGN OF THE SECTOR PROGRAM

Lending instrument: The operation is called a Sector Investment Program and the instrument is a technical assistance loan (TAL). As stated in the PAD, the SIP approach "captures the essential principles on which the ESSP was developed; a sector-wide policy approach and close collaboration between the Government and donors in the preparation of the program."

Consideration was given to the use of an adaptable program loan approach (APL). This would have included basic education as a first phase, followed by technical-vocational training, and higher education. However, it was not adopted because this phasing "would have required defining the total investment for the sub-sectors in the second phase and committing IDA to a specific level of contribution in the investment program." Commitments to specific levels of funding for TVET and higher education were considered premature.

SECTOR PROGRAM CHARACTERISTICS

The ESSP is sector-wide in terms of the agreement between government and donors on the priorities for allocation of resources and the main thrust of the strategy at the different levels of education. The decision to limit the ESSP to basic education at this stage was because of the absence of detailed strategies and programs for the other two subsectors. The overall cost of the program and its financing is included in the Medium-Term Expenditure Framework (MTEF), and was agreed upon by all stakeholders. This is the basis on which donors agreed to share the costs of the program.

Decentralization of the management of education is one of the key objectives of GOM's strategy and this is based on gradually empowering schools and communities to participate in the provision of education. This includes support of school communities through training and transfer of resources. MINED has decided to limit long-term TA to very few key positions, e.g., financial management until suitable staff can be trained and appointed into the regular civil service.

RATIONALE FOR THE SECTOR PROGRAM

With 18 other donors and multiple NGOs implementing more than 150 projects in the sector, the Government and donors saw the dire need to enhance the coordination and impact of projects in the sector. The sector program was fundamentally prepared to overcome weaknesses in the traditional project-based approach. The fragmentation in the use of resources and lack of coordination often led to inefficiency. The MOE decided to adopt a sector approach as a process for more effective

---

[2] UNDP, UNV, UNICEF, WFP, UNFPA, UN Womens Guild.

[3] IDA (World Bank) and ADB.

[4] Catholic Church, EU, etc.

management of funds. Through this integrated SWAP approach, the Government would be better able to increase its effectiveness in the use of domestic and external resources. The SWAP has also forced the transfer of implementation responsibilities from the PIU (GEPE) to the line directorates of the ministry at the central, provincial, and district levels. The resulting decentralization of resources and management responsibilities has also highlighted the need to strengthen the ministry at all levels for more effective operations at a sustained level. This is being addressed in the context of the capacity building program. Success in effective operations at all levels would enhance MINED's capacity to absorb increased resources from the GOM budget and donors. This would be particularly relevant in the context of the HIPC debt relief initiative.

PRECONDITIONS

The preconditions for starting development of a sector-wide approach were as follows: (1) macroeconomic stability; (2) existence of a comprehensive sector development strategy, and (3) government commitment to a sector approach. Soon after the peace agreement sound macroeconomic policies led to unprecedented economic growth and fiscal stability. Improved economic management and stability was facilitated by the development of a comprehensive MTEF. With the MTEF as a back drop GOM developed a coherent sector strategy, and subsequently a coordinated framework that included national and donor agencies for the implementation of programs in the sector. This in turn has reinforced MINED's ownership and control of the process. Although the capacity for a SWAP was not in place at the inception, the government initiated an aggressive capacity development program, which helped create the minimum conditions for completing the preparation of the program and starting implementation. Government's commitment to the process is evidenced by the decision to subsume all projects in the sector within the strat-

egy and the implementation framework agreed for ESSP.

DEFINITION OF THE SECTOR

The sector as defined within ESSP includes primary and secondary general education, technical education and vocational training, and higher education subsectors. The Ministry of Education is responsible for the three subsectors of primary and secondary education, higher education, and technical education vocational training (TEVT), although higher education has some autonomy in management. Some ministries also run training programs independently of MINED. The development of strategies for higher education is, however, the official responsibility of the Ministry of Education. It is done under the aegis of MINED, including preparation of TORs and budgets and task teams appointed by the Minister of Education. With regard to TEVT, MINED coordinates its activities with other Ministries such as Labor and the private sector to avoid conflict in approaches and complementarity during implementation.

PROGRAM LEADERSHIP AND DONOR COORDINATION

The structure for implementing the ESSP is as follows:

* *Program oversight and policy guidance:* The existing coordinating and advisory body of MINED, the Conselho Consultivo do Ministério, will be responsible for policy guidance. The CC comprises the Minister, the Vice-Minister, the Permanent Secretary, and the heads of all national directorates and departments.
* *Organizational structure at the center:* The guiding principle for implementing this program is that the Government will implement the program with existing structures

of the Ministry of Education. The overall structure for implementation proposed is as follows:

(i)   A *Steering Committee* (Comité Paritário de Acompanhamento, COPA) will be the main vehicle for ensuring donor co-ordination and for monitoring and evaluating implementation progress of the ESSP. The committee is headed by the Minister of Education and its members represent key ministries and external partners.

(ii)   A *Technical Committee* (TC) of the ministry will deal with technical issues. The TC will be headed by the Vice-Minister and composed of national directors, the chairs of the working groups, and qualified individuals nominated by the Minister. The Executive Secretary will also be a member of the TC. No donors will be represented on this committee.

(iii)   *Working Groups* (WGs) will be responsible for dealing with technical issues related to the various components, including the preparation of technical papers, annual work plans, annual review of implementation, and advice on changes in the design or policies related to the various components.

(iv)   A *Secretariat*, composed of an Executive Secretary and a few support staff, will provide administrative services to the COPA, TC, and WGs in coordinating and monitoring implementation of the program, including day-to-day donor coordination.

(v)   A *Financial Management Committee* (reporting to the TC) will review quarterly program management reports produced by MINED's Department of Finance and Administration (DAF). The report will cover finances, outputs, and procurement.

❖   *The formal decree for establishing this structure was approved in August 1998.*

❖   *Organizational structure in the provinces and districts.* MINED will phase in decentralization gradually. Decentralization will start with 3 districts out of 10 in the first year, and expand as capacity is built in the regions and regulations for their operations are established. This process will include the development of clear procedures for operations and staff training.

❖   *Donor Coordination:* Donor coordination is led by the Swedish Government. Regular meetings are held to discuss common issues and to promote increased collaboration. A code of conduct has been established to guide donor behavior. When necessary donors meet in smaller groups to discuss specific issues which may not be of interest to the whole community.

PROGRAM DEVELOPMENT

The key milestones in program development included the following: (i) The "National Education Policy and Strategies for Implementation" (NEPS) which was prepared over a two-year period by the Government with some support from external consultants and financing approved by Parliament in 1995, and (ii) The first draft of PEE (Plano Estrategico de Educacao) was prepared, and was discussed at all levels of the Ministry and with donors and civil society over the 1997/98 period. It was endorsed by donors in April 1998. During these consultations the PEE was revised and expanded to include detailed chapters on strategies for teacher training, gender, textbooks, institutional capacity, and school construction. Internal efficiency and cost-effectiveness of the system was also a major concern. MINED refined the strategy to ensure that plans for expanding the system did not prejudice quality. The Council of Ministers approved the strategy in 1998. Following endorsement of the PEE in 1998, the MOE started preparation of the sector program (ESSP). It was recognized that the ESSP would be limited to basic education in the absence of a comprehensive sector analysis of the costs and financing of education, including estimates of returns to higher levels of education and an assessment of the external efficiency of the system. But the program would support the development of the subsector.

LEVEL OF SECTOR ANALYSIS

A number of sector studies were carried out: Public Expenditure Review (1997) by the World Bank, Financial Plan of the ESSP 1997-2001 (1998) by a WB consultant, Teacher Education Reform Proposal (1998) by UNICEF and GOM, Reinforcing Institutional Capacity at MOE (1998) by MOE, World Bank and SIDA, National Policy on Textbooks and Learning Materials (1998) by SIDA and MOE, Mainstreaming Gender in the ESSP 1997-2001 (1998) by UNICEF and MOE, Financial Management Review (1998) by the World Bank. In addition, a number of sector papers were prepared by some donors and MOE on curriculum development, human resource development, and poverty. These studies were revised and built on by the various working groups as the program was finalized.

The economic sector work that was done during preparation was more like a public expenditure review, which was used as a basis for projecting the future growth of the sector on some assumed unit costs. Although the study made some policy recommendations, the analytical underpinnings of the proposed strategy were not clear. The study also did not deal in sufficient depth with issues related to allocation of resources among and within subsectors, or with the internal and operational efficiency of the system. Gender, socioeconomic, and geographic inequities in the provision and in educational attainment were also not fully addressed. The costs of construction were also very high, and the proposed solutions met with stiff resistance from the government because NGOs were permitted to compete for construction contracts as private firms, and because the school designs were considered inappropriate.

Because of gaps in the review of public expenditures a separate study was needed on costs and financing to analyze the education sector from the macro and micro perspectives. The study would focus on demand and supply issues, access, quality, internal and external efficiency, equity, unit costs and cost effectiveness, allocation of resources in the sector and incidence of costs, and management of the system, including decentralization and community participation. This would form the basis for refining the strategy on basic education and for developing detailed strategies for technical education and vocational training, and higher education.

The costs and financing study was not completed prior to appraisal because the PER was considered adequate for a "bridging operation," which was being proposed at the time instead of a SWAP. The processing timetable and resources did not permit the preparation of the costs and financing study when it was decided that a SWAP would be more appropriate. At the same time, the political momentum was there to move forward.

INSTRUMENTS FOR AGREEMENTS

The instruments included aide memoires from the joint MOE-donor meetings; the joint review meeting of the PEE in April 1997, the program pre-appraisal held in September 1997 and the first Joint Annual Review held in May 1998. Consensus was reached on the process and steps to follow, and a code of conduct was developed and agreed to by all.

INSTITUTIONAL CAPACITY

Individual assessments were carried out by external assistance, and MOE set up a task force to prepare the institutional assessment. Three key sector studies were prepared, including one assessment of the financial management system.

A systematic approach to the institutional development of MINED was initiated in 1995, with assistance from various donors, to strengthen the management capacity of the Ministry especially in a number of critical areas. These initiatives were important following the war, which disrupted activities in most parts of the country, and given the generally limited number of qualified people in the country. This effort has been supported by Bank operations in Mozambique, especially the Capacity Building Project, which is supporting secondary and higher education to provide a pool of qualified people to manage the civil service and the private sector. This is especially important for MINED, which needs to manage an expanding program in a rapidly growing economy, and which is also gradually decentralizing management of the sector to the provinces and districts to improve efficiency in the delivery of services. The policies and measures introduced over this period were based on a global assessment of current management practices and capability, including operational procedures and methods. This assessment, as well as the development and implementation of the program was conducted using a participatory approach. This has resulted in ownership and an identification with the objectives and activities by staff at all levels in MINED. MINED plans to build on this foundation by conducting a more thorough analysis of each administrative unit of the Ministry at the central, provincial, and district levels, as a basis for defining the capacity needed in each section and at each level for efficient delivery of quality education.

The methodology to be used in performing this institutional assessment is based on an operational definition of capacity. Applying this definition, the capacity of all the organizations involved in the implementation of the proposed program will be analyzed by focusing on organization, leadership, financial resources, material resources, human resources, and work practices. The assessment team will focus first on the question "What needs to be done in order to implement the program?" or "For what is capacity required?" It will then determine "Who needs to do it?" or "Whose capacity within the education sector is in question?"

Answering these two questions, the team will systematically identify all the organizations, and the organizational units, that are to be involved in the implementation of the proposed investment program. Once these are identified, the team will examine the five factors indicated above with respect to each and every organization and organizational unit individually. This examination will help determine institutional weaknesses and capacity gaps.

Four types of alternative capacity building measures will then be considered in each case where a capacity gap is identified:

- ❖ To change practices, ways of doing things and procedures, where such a change can improve the capacity of the organization or unit involved, without having to allocate it more resources.
- ❖ To allocate, or reallocate, financial and human resources for the performance of certain activities, where the gaps are considered to be the result of inadequate resources.
- ❖ To spread certain activities over a longer period of time, or to reduce the scope of certain development objectives, where additional capacity is required but cannot be built immediately, or during the currently scheduled implementation period.
- ❖ To follow a certain mix of these three alternatives.

The institutional assessment team will consist of members of the working group on capacity building and a long-term consultant from ASDI, supported by a Bank Team. The officials and the consultant will be trained to apply the methodology. By the end of this assessment, they will be able to use the methodology to carry out similar assessments independently. The managers of each organization and unit assessed will be thoroughly briefed on the objectives of the capacity building initiative, as well as the methodology, and will take an active part in the assessment and identification of solutions.

STAKEHOLDER CONSULTATION

During the preparation of the PEE and of the ESSP program, the MOE organized wide-ranging discussions at central, provincial, district, school, and community levels. As stated in the PAD, "The Government's Strategic Plan was developed with the participation of a full range of stakeholders including parents, local communities, employers, NGOs and religious organizations. This was achieved through: (a) bringing teachers and staff into the decision-making process through various working groups, (b) increasing representation of actors at the provincial, district and school levels in the planning process, (c) strengthening pedagogical support zones and training school directors to interact more effectively with communities, and (d) holding consultative sessions with civil society" (PAD, pp. 30-31). Overall the ESSP program is perceived to have been "prepared and owned by the Mozambicans."

THE SECTOR PROGRAM

Objectives and Strategy

The objective of the ESSP is to achieve increased and equitable access to higher quality education through improvement in the management of education in order to promote social and economic development.

Content

The ESSP includes four components: (1) Quality of primary education: training and pedagogical support for teachers, curriculum revision, increased supply of learning materials, strengthening of student assessment and examinations, direct grant support to schools, and training of school directors. (2) Access to basic education: building and rehabilitation of schools; promotion of girls' education; development of non-formal education; and pilot programs for special education. (3) Strengthening MOE Institutional Capacity: strengthened organi-

zational structure of the MOE and support to decentralization; development of MOE policy and planning; building MOE financial management; and conduct of monitoring and evaluation. (4) TVET: production of a subsector strategy and financing its implementation. (PAD, Annex 2 provides a detailed description of the program.)

Organization and Management

The guiding principle for implementing the program is that the Government will implement the program within existing structures of the MOE (PAD: 14). Also see previous discussion of this subject.

Financing

The estimated cost of the ESSP including contingencies is US$717.2 million. As a comprehensive plan for the sector, the ESSP includes the costs of salaries (US$293) and other recurrent costs including operation and maintenance. Of total costs, the Government would finance an estimated US$ 444.6 million, NGOs US$ 30.0 million, communities (in kind or in cash) US$ 5.0 million, IDA US$ 71 million, and other donors US$ 118.8 million.

Modus Operandi

Monitoring and evaluation arrangements: MINED will monitor and evaluate the program within the structure setup for implementation and using detailed terms of reference for key units within this structure. Monitoring and outcome *indicators* will allow MINED to measure progress and will form the basis for joint supervision with other donors. Each unit involved with implementation will develop instruments for monitoring its respective component, while the Planning Unit and the DAF will consolidate and analyze statistical, financial, and physical data on the rate of implementation. A system will be introduced to provide information on output indicators such as expenditures, units built, and number of teachers trained. Capacity will be built in the provinces for collecting monitoring data. The Executive Secretary (responsible to the Technical Committee and CC) will synthesize the results. The donor group will coordinate and manage donor-related matters, such as the preparation of statements of donor contributions, to minimize MINED's time-consuming task of dealing with individual donors.

Formalized *supervision* will take place twice a year to review progress in implementation. Government and donors will jointly prepare the terms of reference and participate in the mission. The Government and each of the provinces will prepare annual *progress reports* that not only assess overall progress but also highlight components or districts with bottlenecks or weak performance. MINED's information-gathering activities will be the basis of the reporting requirements for the *joint annual review* meetings with donors. This review will be carried out immediately following MINED's annual meeting with provincial and district directors. The first annual review was held in May 1999. A *midterm evaluation* of the program will be held no later than 30 months after program effectiveness, in accordance with terms of reference agreed upon by MINED and the donor community.

Monitoring indicators: As part of the ESSP a program monitoring reporting system (PMR) will be developed to monitor education outcomes, financial indicator and link expenditures, and outputs and schedule of implementation, including procurement, for each component. Currently the following indicators have been identified:

(1) Increased proportion of students passing key primary and secondary examinations:
  (i)   Grade 5 from 54% to 75%
  (ii) Grade 7 from 37% to 60%
  (iii) Grade 10 from 33% to 55%
(2) A reduction in the average repetition and dropout rates by half for primary and lower secondary.
(3) An increase in gross enrollment rates (i) Grades 1-5 from 67% to 86%; and (ii) Grades 6-7 from 15% to 30%.

(4) An increase in enrollment in the schools and districts where classrooms are built, equivalent to about 75% of new capacity created.
(5) Implementation of at least 80% of the work program for each year measured by the physical targets and budget spent for program and routine activities.
(6) Achievement of the agreed rate of decentralization of management to the provinces and districts as defined in the Program Implementation Manual.

In addition to these six indicators agreed to by all donors, consensus was reached during the first annual meeting to expand the indicators to include: (i) increases in girls' enrollment and retention, (ii) improvement in learning outcomes (EFA indicator #15), and (iii) improvement in completion rates at all levels. Independent consultants will also carry out technical audits of the program starting in the second year to assess the quality of implementation and make recommendations for improvement (PAD, p. 19). Procurement under the program will be decentralized to the provinces, although this process is still at an initial stage. The center will carry out all ICB procurement and consultant selection under the program, coordinate all activities at the provincial level, and assist the provinces with standard bid documents, construction plans, and technical advice. To strengthen the center's performance, an experienced executive secretary has been appointed, staff from GEPE (the former project implementation unit) have been incorporated into MINED central functions, and an advanced procurement course was held in March 1999 in Maputo.

At the provincial level, only three pilot provinces will manage their own procurement in the first year of the program. Each of the provinces will establish program implementation arrangements based in the provincial MINED offices, supported through capacity building. The provincial MINED office will implement the procurement of small works, furniture, and educational materials using National Competitive Bidding (NCB) and will assist rural districts to utilize community participation in school construction. The MINED offices will be encouraged to delegate management and supervision of works to more experienced local consulting firms. A detailed list of actions to be taken by central and provincial MINED offices prior to program implementation have been agreed on.

Financial Monitoring

MINED's Directorate of Administration and Finance (DAF) will be responsible for overall management and reporting of the principal financial resources for the ESSP. Every quarter, the Financial Management Committee (reporting to the Technical Committee) will review DAF's program management report. Independent auditors acceptable to IDA will audit program accounts annually and provide a management letter that recommends improvements to the financial management system. In the medium to long term, the Government proposes to introduce a new financial management system (FMS), as part of the overall civil service reform program.

Harmonization of Donors' Procurement Procedures

Harmonization of procurement and disbursement procedures is feasible under the Program and has been the subject of a detailed study by IDA. It is expected that some of the donors will agree on common thresholds for procurement under NCB; the use of post-review and of reporting formats. Donors may also agree on the use of standard documents and procedures for advertising, evaluating, and awarding the contracts. IDA procedures and documentation will be followed for all ICB procurement.

GOM procurement regulations may be used for NCB contracts, provided that IDA procurement regulations would prevail in case of conflict.

Financing

Within the five-year ESSP program of US$717 million, IDA will maintain a presence in strategic components. The financing plan for the program was drafted during the joint donor assessment mission in May 1998 and further refined during appraisal in late 1998. By appraisal a total of about US$85 million had been committed to ESSP by various donors to support ongoing activities that were part of the program. Approximately US$105 million was also expected to be provided by donors over the five-year program period. The schedule for agreement on new funds would follow the natural cycles of the various agencies. A number of donors also (e.g., Denmark, the Netherlands, Sweden, Ireland, and the United Kingdom/DFID) planned to provide part of their funding for the program through direct budgetary support. Some donors even tied all new funding to agreement on budgetary support by at least a core group of donors. About US$70 million was expected to be provided through this means. The Bank was the donor of last resort, but became involved in a core strategic program because of the uncertainty over when (and perhaps whether) new funding would materialize from several key donors. The normal approval cycles for the various donors meant that commitment of new funding would be drawn out over two or three years. Conditioning assistance on budget support added more fragility to the equation. Budget support was entirely new. No one knew how to do it. The Bank therefore agreed to participate in the financing of several components.[5] Core

---

[5] In-service teacher training (US$6 million), pedagogical support for teachers through Zips (US$6.1 million), curriculum transformation (US$1.0 million), learning materials (US$6.4 million), examinations (US$0.30 million), direct support to schools (US$4.9 million), training of school directors (US$1.0 million), school construction and rehabilitation (US$31.8 million), gender initiatives (US$5 million), and capacity building (US$8.3 million), for a total of US$70.8 million. A small amount of funds will also be allocated for developing strategies for further development of technical education and vocational training.

financing by the Bank was designed to ensure continued financing of the program as a whole pending the release of other donor funding. There is agreement between the Government and donors that nothing outside the strategic framework will be financed during the period of program implementation. The Bank disburses on the basis of incurred eligible expenditures included in the annual revised targets (annual work plans) through the Special Account.

Administration, Accounting, Financial Management, and Auditing Functions

MINED's Directorate of Administration and Finance (DAF) will be responsible for overall management and reporting of the principal financial resources for the ESSP. The Government will keep the funds from IDA and each other donor in separate accounts but will move toward common procurement, financial management, and auditing procedures acceptable to all partners. Financial statements will show ESSP basket expenditures as well as the source of the funds. Donor agencies support the *gradual* transfer of funds to MINED through budget support as its financial management capacities improve. In the medium to long term, the Government proposes to introduce a new financial management system (FMS), as part of the overall civil service reform program.

Conditionality

The program was designed to be consistent with the Government's Medium Term Expenditure Framework and the targets set out under the ESSP. In the Government's Letter of Sector Policy and the attached policy matrix the detailed qualitative and financial indicators and Government conditions are stipulated, including increasing government budget for education from 18.2% in 1998 to 21% in 2003 (from 3.5% to about 5% of GDP). In addition the share of basic education will be increased by up to 2% of GNP in the same period. On the qualitative side the targets

were agreed to as outlined under the previous section on monitoring. It was further agreed that no new project would be initiated outside the agreed framework. More specifically, several process-related conditions are incl uded, such as joint annual program reviews in May, submission of annual work program and budget by October, submission of semi-annual progress reports including outcome and performance indicators. Other conditions are related to the preparation of specific plans (e.g., community involvement in establishing and running schools, policy and plan for privatization of textbook publication, plan for improvement of internal efficiency, plan for management of direct grants for schools, and plan for improving time on task in schools). As the program is integrated into the Ministry and later, the annual work plans discussed widely, it guarantees consistency; and any issue that comes up should be resolved during this process.

IMPLEMENTATION OF THE SECTOR PROGRAM

Implementation Experience

The IDA Credit became effective on August 3, 1999 and implementation is still in its early stages. In the first year of the ESSP the Government focused on setting up the financial and institutional arrangements for the ESSP. Preparation of the comprehensive provincial plans were the main focus during this period. The new organizational structure has shown to be an efficient structure for implementing the program as evidenced by the following: (i) coordination among national directors has increased, (ii) integration of the program in MINED has improved, (iii) transparency in the use of donor funds has increased, and (iv) the government is becoming increasingly proactive in managing implementation because of the realization that it is accountable for results.

Commitments of some donor funds were linked to budget support, (consistent with the spirit of ESSP) with the expectation that this would be easy to arrange. This turned out not to be the case. A joint-donor mission for the education sector assessed the scope for using this approach in September, and recommended against it because of capacity concerns at MINED and MPF. Subsequently, the Swedish, Irish, and Dutch aid agencies proposed the pooling of funds at the MINED level until the concerns regarding the flow of funds through the MPF were addressed. The Bank decided to join this group, and the mechanism for doing this is now being explored. The joint financial management mission in which consultants from Irish Aid, SIDA, Dfid, CIDA, Finnida, and the World Bank participated, and which was led by MOE, is a good example of the new collaboration among partners.

There has been little or no disagreement over strategy. Donors have been willing to use the implementation designs agreed by the MINED and collaboration is strong at this level.

Main Achievements

Although tangible education results can only be measured over the long term, there is clear evidence that the ESSP has proven itself to be an efficient vehicle for moving the program forward; it has strengthened government ownership, it has empowered national directorates and ministry staff, and the program has been integrated into the ministry increasing transparency and ensuring increased effectiveness in the implementation of agreed activities. The reinforcement of the authority of national directors has given them the authority over externally financed activities, including IDA-funded activities. While it was agreed at the first annual review that the move toward common procedures is a longer-term effort, a joint framework–joint collaboration in assessing needs and requirements to move the process forward for establishing common financial and procurement procedures is already under way. This rationalization is further exemplified in the joint work and missions being undertaken.

The main factor explaining the success of the SWAP is government ownership and strong government leadership.

- ❖ Agreement of so many (18) donors on a common, single program.
- ❖ Harmonization of monitoring & evaluation procedures, including common indicators, common reporting, joint annual reviews, etc.
- ❖ "Institutionalizing" the program, by moving the locus of control from separate and isolated PIUs into the main offices and departments of the MOE.

Main Problems (or lack of achievements) Design Phase

There were no major disagreements or misunderstanding during the design phase. There was some concern about the ability of the government to train and finance the required number of teachers required for expansion. When this was analyzed in detail, especially in light of the much lower population figures from the recent census and plans to improve internal efficiency, this turned out to be less of an issue. There were similar concerns about other issues, but these were also resolved following further analysis.

During implementation: There have been no unexpected problems during the implementation period. Concerns and issues have been expressed early on and have been discussed and resolved in the spirit of collaboration and mutual professional respect.

OBSERVATIONS AND POSSIBLE LESSONS

The following lessons can be drawn from the development of the ESSP Sector Program in education:

- ❖ *Conditions for the Development of a SWAP:*
  (1) The experience with the sector program in Mozambique shows the importance of: (i) starting with a Government-prepared strategy in which donors play a supporting role; (ii) government tak-

ing the leadership in coordinating the donors; (iii) setting up clear institutional arrangements and an organization structure for collaboration within the ministry and with and among donors at the very beginning, especially during the preparation of the policy and strategy, as this in turn sets the stage for the future; and (iv) building consensus at all levels of government and related institutions, as well as among stakeholders such as civil society, NGOs, and private institutions.

(2) The initial step for launching a sector program is a coherent strategy under which all stakeholders will operate. The move toward budget support and common procedures should not be an objective by itself, but a natural development toward building national capacity.

❖ *Benefits of a SWAP*
   (1) A Government-led SWAP focuses attention on country priorities instead of supply-driven agendas.
   (2) A SWAP reinforces the Government's control over funds, especially external financing, minimizing the margin for individual donor negotiations and donor-driven agendas, thereby increasing the effectiveness in policy execution (funds spent on activities for which they are intended and in consistency with national development objectives and priorities).
   (3) A SWAP increases Government accountability as its authority over activities and funding increases, thereby, increasing stakes and commitment.
   (4) A SWAP eases the administrative burden of Government in dealing with multiple different donors and systems
   (5) A SWAP demands the development of capacity and national systems, instead of individual and parallel systems.

❖ *Common Procedures under a SWAP:*
   (1) There is a need to revise government's procurement procedures to ensure that it satisfies donor demands for efficiency, competition and transparency in the award of contracts. This would obviate the need for the tortuous attempt to harmonize donor policies.
   (2) Donors need to understand better and be involved with the evolution of changes in public financial management, especially relating to changes in the budget law to help design systems that will satisfy the needs for transparency and accountability.

❖ *Precondition and When Not to Do a SWAP*
   (1) The starting point of a SWAP should be based on Government desire and commitment to move toward an integrated strategy and sector program. If government commitment is not there, the coalition of donors would be fragile and eventually break down at some point.
   (2) A clearly costed program consistent with a Medium-Term Expenditure Framework would constitute the major condition for initiating a SWAP process.

❖ *Risks*
   (1) Some of the risks concern the enormous amount of time spent on donor coordination with limited concrete output. This is especially the case if there is insistence on budget support and the use of common procedures at the inception of the program. Capacity building should be seen as one of the objectives of the SWAP.

❖ *Sector Performance*
   (1) A set of indicators should be adopted on sector performance. A Financial Committee should be established to monitor performance and match expenditures with activities. These data should be included in a comprehensive monitoring and evaluation mechanism.

List of "dos" and "don'ts" for SWAP design and implementation.

(A) Do: It is important to agree in advance on ground rules for all parties. It is difficult to keep a diverse group of donors together. There will be disagreements, which means that procedures need to be agreed in advance on how to handle disagreements. Government needs to take the lead.

(B) Do: Specifically, the role and authority of the "lead donor" should be clarified in advance.

(C) Do: The sector program depends to an extraordinary extent on the collaborative relations established between the parties, that—in turn—depends on openness. It means, inter alia, the Government has to be committed to a process of examining itself as well as donors putting aside disagreements.

(D) Don't: The ultimate objective is not harmonization of donor procedures, but development of good government systems.

(E) Do: Financing the core program – does this approach reduce the risk and uncertainty that some donors may not contribute? No, it means that the Government will be able to deliver its education services with a view to ensuring long term improvements.

(F) Do: Joint annual reviews—what do they need to be successful? Government needs to take the lead, otherwise the annual review runs the risk of representing individual donor agendas.

(G) Do: Monitoring indicators—how should they be improved? With the development of internal capacity and systems. It is important to note that monitoring indicators are not only statistical, but the overall performance of the sector can be reinforced through adequate institutional setup.

TABLE 1
1786 – Mozambique, Gen. Educ. Sec. Exp. Program
Project Status Report Date: **5/20/99**

Region:	AFR	Country:	MOZAMBIQUE			Sector:	EP	Lending Instr:	TAL
Prg Obj Cat:	PA	EA Cat:	C	PTI?	Y	NGO?	N	Resettlement?	N

LOAN INFORMATION

Agree Type	L/C/G No.	Orig Amt	Rev'd Amt	Currency Indicator	Prod Line	Signing Date	Effective Date	Suppl Prj ID
IDA	31720	51.10 (SDR)			PE	3/4/99		

Total Original Amount (SDR):	51.10	Total Revised Amount (SDR):	0.00

COFINANCING INFORMATION

Agency		Board Amount ($M)	Current Amount ($M)
	Total	0.00	0.00

	Guarantee Type:		Guarantee Amount ($M):	

This form is part of: **Initial Summary**
Read together with:

( ) Aide-memoire	Mission End Date:		This Form PSR Date:	5/20/99
( ) BTO memo of:	Months since last mission:		Last Form PSR Date:	
( ) Follow-up letter of:	Next mission planned:			

SUPERVISION EFFORT	Total Staff-Weeks	Total $000	Field Staff-Weeks	Field $000	As of 5/20/99
Current FY - Planned	12.60	38.48			
Current FY - Actual	26.38	89.97	1.13	4.43	
Board through preceding FY	0.00	0.00	0.00	0.00	
Total Actual	26.38	89.97	1.13	4.43	

UPI No.	Mission Member	Division	No. of Fld Days	Role or Specialization	Previous Mission

Zambia Education Case Study[1]
Basic Education Subsector Investment Program (BESSIP)

BACKGROUND

Reflecting economic deterioration, Zambia's education system also deteriorated significantly during the 1980s. A new administration with a different economic philosophy came into power in 1991, and embarked on the process of articulating its policies in a number of sectors, including education. This led eventually to the issuance of a Government policy document, "Educating Our Future: National Policy on Education." The Policy was adopted by Parliament in 1996. The document identifies the problems facing the sector, identifies targets for 2005 and 2015, and highlights a strategy for moving forward. At the time, the education sector was beset with myriad problems: Two of the key issues are stagnating enrollment rates and poor learning outcomes. These problems leave the low share of government budget allocated to education and a misallocation of education within to tertiary education—in large part for student personal welfare. The effectiveness of teaching in basic education is compromised by limited instructional times, inappropriate language of instruction in rural areas, inadequately prepared and motivated teachers, lack of instructional materials, the poor state of classrooms, and inadequate programs to help disadvantaged children. Support

from external donors has been fragmented. Despite considerable external support, Zambia's education indicators have stagnated. The trend suggested the need for a different approach so as to make a bigger impact on solving pressing educational issues. Already in Zambia two other sector-wide approaches were under implementation, in agriculture and health. The government and donor community were familiar with the approach and its potential benefits. It was only natural, then, that the Government and all major donors decided to try a sector-wide approach.

THE BESSIP PROGRAM

The Basic Education Sub-sector Investment Program (BESSIP) is the national program of basic education of the Government, developed between 1996-98. The two main objectives are to increase enrollment and to improve learning outcomes. Gross enrollment ratios are planned to increase from 84% at present to 100% by 2005, and net enrollment ratios to 90%. Improved learning outcomes are also the focus and will be measured by national assessments. The Program includes eight components: instructional materials, teacher development and

---

[1] This case study is based on interviews with the two Task Team Leaders, Mr. Paud Murphy and Mr. Bruce Jones, and the following two documents: IDA Project Appraisal Document, March 5, 1999, No. 19008ZA, and Barbara Chilangwa, "Issues, Experiences, Challenges and Lessons in the Process of Establishing the Zambian Basic Education Sub-Sector Investment Programme (BESSIP)".

deployment, school health and nutrition, equity, infrastructure, curriculum development, capacity building and decentralization, and BESSIP program management.

SWAP DESIGN

Lending instrument: BESSIP is supported by an adaptable program loan (APL). The overall program is five and a half years. The first phase is from January 1999 to June 2002, to which IDA is contributing US$40 million. A second phase is expected from July 2001 to June 2006 including US$60 million in IDA financing. Both phases focus on basic education, with more emphasis on capacity building in the first phase and pilot measures to increase enrollments and learning outcomes for disadvantaged groups. Key triggers for starting the second phase are: (1) at least 20.5% of government discretionary budget (the portion of the budget available for annual allocation through the budgetary process, but excluding the portion of the budget committed to debt service and pensions as a consequence of budgetary decisions of earlier years) allocated to the Ministry of Education and maintenance of at least 60% share of the MOE budget for primary schools, (2) share of trained teachers increased in rural schools; (3) construction of 2000 classrooms; (4) bursary scheme in place for poor children; (5) completion and publishing of results of a first national assessment of learning achievements; and (6) district education boards established and functioning in 60% of districts – as well as preparation of the second phase.

Rationale for the SWAP: Zambia has considerable experience with external financing in education. About 14 external agencies have provided support to the education sector. Much of the support has been fragmented, with each project having its own institutional arrangements. Despite considerable external support, Zambia's education indicators have stagnated. The trend suggested the need for a different approach so as to make a bigger impact on solving pressing educational issues. Already in Zambia two other sector-wide approaches were under imple-

mentation, in agriculture and health. The government and donor community were familiar with the approach and its potential benefits. It was only natural, then, that government and all major donors decided to try a sector-wide approach involving a common sector policy framework and medium term investment program as well as promoting Government capacity and leadership.

SWAP characteristics: The coverage of the program is not sector-wide, but it nevertheless has most of the characteristics of a SWAP. It stems from an overall policy on education and training, "Educating Our Future—1996". It is based on a long-term vision and program for the top priority subsector, basic education, on which the Government and all major donors agree. There is an agreed expenditure framework for the subsector program. Local stakeholders were in charge of development of the program, particularly after a new Minister of Education took over (see below). All the main donors have agreed to finance a share of the costs of the program. Finally, efforts have been made to use normal Government capacity and processes and adopt common procedures and reporting as far as possible to minimize administrative burdens on the Government.

Preconditions: Several preconditions were considered to be essential before embarking on a modified sector-wide approach. First was relative macroeconomic stability, so that resource allocations could be planned with some degree of certainty. (Unfortunately, macroeconomic stability has not yet been achieved in Zambia. The rate of inflation has recently been about 30%.) Second, a conceptual framework existed for the whole sector in the form of the 1996 National Education Policy. Third, most donors supported the development of a broad program approach in view of frustrations with success of previous projects. Finally, there was strong Government leadership—not at the start of the process but that emerged and allowed the program approach to flourish.

Definition of the sector: Development of the program went through several stages of reduction in scope to achieve a final definition of the "sector," or in this case, "sub-sector." Initially an attempt was made at developing a comprehensive Education Sector Investment Program (ESIP), coordinated by an ESIP Secretariat. Higher education was excluded from the beginning on the basis that it was an area of lower priority for new investment, than basic education and training. ESIP still included four ministries, (i) the Ministry of Education; (ii) Science Technology and Vocational Training; (iii) Youth, Sport and Child Development, and (iv) Community Development and Social Services.) In September 1997 the Government agreed with donors for its agenda in the education and training sector to be supported by two financing packages, one for basic education (BESSIP) and another for training (TSSIP). BESSIP is led by the Ministry of Education, and the great majority of its activities are within MOE. However, a bursaries subcomponent will be administered through the Public Welfare Assistance Scheme of MCDSS, and a Microprojects Unit outside MOE (attached to the Ministry of Finance and Economic Development) will continue to administer community-implemented school construction activities.

Program leadership: After the former Vice President became Minister of Education in December 1997, he convened a conference with donors in February 1998 and gave his clear vision and authority for the development of a sector program. This was a seminal event in the development of BESSIP because it gave potential donors a clear impression of government leadership of the process and clarity about program goals and content.

Donor coordination: On the donor side, the Bank had been financing, through a Japanese grant, the studies under the ESIP. Donor coordination for BESSIP was achieved through an informal donors group, the "Consultative Forum" for meetings convened periodically by the ESIP Secretariat. Since then, an electronic forum of BESSIP donors has been established with continuous communications through e-mail. In early stages some donors expressed concern over the perceived "dominant role of the World Bank". During the past year, this concern diminished as MOE displayed increased ownership of the program, and as three of the bilaterals (DfID, USAID, and NORAD) added education specialists to their Lusaka offices specifically for BESSIP, enabling them to play a greater role in the dialogue. Close donor collaboration is evident in the fact that four other donors served as observers (and often participated in discussions) at negotiations of the IDA Credit. However, at about the time of negotiations the Belgian authorities gave Zambia funds for teacher training without any discussion in advance among the donors.

Program development: The first stage in the development of the program was the efforts at development of the ESIP starting in 1994 and the adoption of the National Policy on Education in 1996. During this process some 17 studies were generated on specific issues, of which 11 concerned basic education. These reports generated discussions and fostered mutual understanding about the issues and consensus on the interventions required. All donors were broadly comfortable with the directions in the Policy. However, the Policy needed more specificity on timing and volumes. These were generated through Bank missions on which donors were invited to participate. The culmination was a joint donor appraisal mission in September 1998, which produced a Joint Appraisal Report. By the conclusion of the appraisal process two additional important documents had been produced by the Government, partly with Bank assistance: The Program Implementation Plan (PIP) and the "Statement on Education Policy Implementation during 1999-2002."[2] Basically throughout the process no major disagreements emerged between the Government and donors, or among the donors about the policy aspects of the Program. The Ministry of Education did modify its position to allow more community demand-driven construction administered

---

[2] Officially submitted by the Government to the Bank and appearing as Annex 11 of the Project Appraisal Document. All partners had a chance to comment.

by the Microprojects Unit under the program. Considerable discussion took place, however, concerning implementation and financing under the proposed SWAP. Agreements were reached relatively easily to coordinate and use common procedures/reports on program planning and review, budgeting and performance monitoring, and progress reporting. Most difficult was harmonizing approaches on procurement, contract administration, finance, and accounting. The amount and nature of institutional capacity building needed before investment was always a major topic. Another was the modalities of financial assistance. In particular so much confusion reigned about "basket funding" that the term was banned. The PAD presents a typology that was developed to clarify the various methods of providing financing under BESSIP. (See Financing, below.) However, where one donor was active and heavily involved in certain components (e.g., the Danish program for teacher training), the Bank tended not to enter into a deep dialogue and glossed over differences.

Level of sector analysis: The BESSIP program was not preceded by any formal education sector work. The ESIP had produced about nine documents that provided background information on basic education. In November 1996 a consultant prepared an Education and Training Sector Expenditure Review that also proved to be useful background information. In addition, more than ten studies on specific aspects of basic education were financed through a PHRD grant managed by the BESSIP Secretariat. Topics included equity, health and nutrition, instructional materials, teacher development, construction, and examinations. However, the Secretariat generally did not have the capacity to manage quality in analytical work and the work tended to be almost exclusively by educationists. The results were generally disappointing. At one stage of the review process, for example, criticism was voiced in the Bank that the Program did not have a specific vision for how to proceed to the ultimate objective of universal primary education. Bank missions had to make up for the lack of analytical rigor in the background studies.

Instruments for agreements: The Government produced the basic national education policy document with which donors broadly agreed. In 1996 the donors signed a Joint Statement expressing their interest in supporting education in Zambia through a sectoral approach, but also expressing concern over the low share of the Government budget devoted to the education sector. In 1998 four bilateral donors established a preparatory fund to support the initial activities for BESSIP. The joint appraisal (in which 17 donors participated!) produced a common, joint appraisal report. A sample "code of conduct" prepared by the European Union was circulated. While not officially agreed, it provides a generally accepted statement of principles. Finally, all parties have agreed to the Program Implementation Plan that was reviewed at appraisal and subsequently revised.

Institutional capacity: No formal instruments were used to assess the capacity of the Government to implement the program, and a comprehensive professional analysis was not undertaken. In 1997, a team of officials from the Management Development Division of the Cabinet Office and the Ministry of Education prepared a Report on the Restructuring of the Ministry of Education. The Restructuring Report assigns the responsibilities of District Education Offices to District Education Boards and District Education Standards Officers. At the Headquarters, the Deputy Permanent Secretary posts are abolished, and there are six units whose heads report directly to the Permanent Secretary: Planning and Information; Human Resources and Adminstration; Standards and Curriculum Development; Teacher Education; Accounts; and Procurement. This restructuring was intended to support decentralization, and otherwise enhance the capacity of the Ministry to meet its mandate. However, until now the reforms have not been introduced because of lack of money to compensate those persons whose jobs would be abolished. Considerable attention was devoted to financial management and procurement capacity, and specialists in these fields participated in the appraisal.

Stakeholder consultation: Early in the process of developing the program some stakeholder consultation took place in the preparation and discussion of the various studies under the ESIP. The 1996 National Policy on Education in fact calls for the Government to work closely with NGOs, local communities, donors, and other stakeholders in the provision of education. However, observers of the BESSIP process stated that actually there was only limited participation by teachers' unions, NGOs, and the community school sector in the process of program development. Those occasions that were meant to foster exchanges of ideas tended to be dominated by donors.

Financing: The first phase of BESSIP is expected to cost US$340 million, of which the Government is expected to finance about half, IDA 12%, and other donors 38%, of which about half would be new commitments and the rest ongoing assistance programs. IDA support is structured in such as way as to enable IDA funds to be devoted to any of the components. About three-fourths of the credit proceeds are allocated to specific categories of new expenditure, and one-fourth was left unallocated so as to flexibly meet needs for which the Government is currently seeking grant aid, but not all of which may materialize. Initially funds are likely to finance schools, textbooks, and vehicles and other equipment to support decentralization.

Procurement: Procurement under the IDA Credit will be carried out along traditional lines. A Procurement and Financial Procedures Manual is being finalized which will be used for the IDA Credit, but the Government has solicited suggestions from other donors so that it can be adaptable to support provided by other donors.

Financial flows and disbursements: The BESSIP Preparatory Fund received funds into a common account ("pooling") by several donors, including the U.K., Dutch, Irish, and Norwegian donor agencies. This became the model that Government wished to use for the full program implementation. It was recognized as the ideal method during the joint appraisal, but was not foreseen as being acceptable to most donors because of weaknesses in existing capacity for financial management. Instead, BESSIP was explicitly designed to allow flexibility in the channeling of funds by donors. The following external financing modalities are recognized:

Risks and dangers: Given the broad subsector objectives that the Program seeks to achieve, staff feel that the risks of giving important responsibilities to mainstream MOE units are outweighed by the potential benefits of this approach.

Conditionality: The IDA Credit Agreement refers to the letter from the Minister of Finance dated February 15, 1999, with attachments, describing "the Program". Article V of the Credit Agreement gives IDA the right to suspend disbursements in the event that "a situation shall have arisen which shall make it improbable that the Program or a significant part thereof will be carried out." A condition of effectiveness is the adoption of an acceptable Procurement and Financial Management Plan. The main assurance is tied to the process of semiannual re-

TABLE 1

Category	Case 1	Case 2	Case 3	Case 4
Funds controlled by:	MOE	MOE	MOE	Donor
Funds available for which components of BESIP?	All	All	Limited number	One or a small number
"Pooling" of funds in common account?	Yes	No	No	No
Examples of donors using each method:	Dutch, Irish	IDA		

Disbursements are made in traditional ways under BESSIP.

views, including approval of the Annual Work Program and Budget for the succeeding year. In one sense, the triggers for Phase Two are expected to be an incentive for good performance under the first phase. Good performance will almost automatically yield additional funding for the second phase. However, the triggers for the second phase are relatively imprecise, leave much to interpretation, and were set at levels the Bank staff are reasonably confident the Government can meet so that funds can be readily disbursed under the program.

SWAP IMPLEMENTATION

Organization and management: Three new groups were established to oversee implementation. (1) Program policy is guided by a Joint Steering Committee (JSC) chaired by the Minister of Education and including MOE staff, cooperating partners, and NGOs. All donors are eligible to attend these meetings. The JSC meets twice a year to review the work of the previous year and plan for the following year. The JSC is supported by a technical committee chaired by the Permanent Secretary, namely, the Program Development Implementation and Monitoring Committee (PIC: Four bilateral donors plus the Bank represent all donors in the work of the PIC. Day-to-day management of the program is through the Management Implementation Team (MIT), including a core team of officials and component managers who are line officials. MIT is chaired by the Deputy Permanent Secretary (Technical Cooperation). In addition, the MIT is supported by five sub-committees covering cross cutting issues such as decentralization, monitoring and evaluation, human resource development and gender.

Modus operandi: The key condition, as stated above, concerns a process of twice-yearly reviews of program implementation. The MOE organizes Semi-Annual Reviews each year. (Note: In addition to the two Semi-Annual Reviews, there may be "special" JSC meetings. For example, there has been a special JSC meeting on HIV/AIDS in relation to BESSIP.) The May meeting reviews accounts and progress on the previous year's work; the November meeting plans work for the next year, including financial projections. The November meeting considers a draft Annual Work Program and Budget for the succeeding year, including an annual procurement plan for goods, works, and services to be financed. Based on actual experience and performance, the sector program can be revised and adapted to new circumstances. For example, the semiannual reviews monitor progress toward achievement of the targeted increase in the percentage of expenditures going to the Ministry of Education, and the maintenance of at least a 60% share for primary schools within the MOE budget.

Implementation experience: The IDA Credit is expected to be declared effective shortly. The delays were caused because the required procurement and financial procedures manual had not yet been accepted. The first semiannual review took place in May 1999 with mixed results. Donors were disappointed in the quality of the Government's progress report. Considerable time was absorbed by the proposal put forward by some bilateral agencies, but not accepted by MOE, that a high-level "management accountant" should be appointed in the Ministry of Education. Not much time was left for monitoring or capacity building. Ultimately, however, the donors were satisfied with the agreements reached at the review.

OUTCOMES SO FAR

Main achievements:

(1) The process of developing the SWAP has forced the Ministry of Education to become more coherent and organized than it was in the past. Previously, different units did not communicate with each other; each unit followed its own course. There was little sense of working toward common objectives. The BESSIP process significantly improved internal communications.

(2) Key people in Government and the donors have learned a great deal about working

together toward common objectives. The objectives of the program are much more widely shared as a result of the process of program development.

(3) A process has been established for dealing with tangential suggestions – although it was not applied in the case of the very late Belgian assistance.

LESSONS

The following lessons should be noted:

(1) There must be a champion for the program with sufficient authority and leadership on the government side. In BESSIP the process foundered for a while because there was no leadership. When the former Vice President became Minister of Education about 18 months ago, the leadership was established

to make the process truly Government-driven. Without a minimum level of leadership, it would be impossible to do a SIP or SWAP.

(2) You cannot engage in too much communication with other donors. Whatever you have done, it is not enough. The corollary to this, of course, is that donor coordination takes time. It has high transaction costs and drives up the task budget.

(3) The program had high-level endorsement. The National Policy on Education had been reviewed and approved by Parliament. This level of approval proved helpful in ensuring support by other Ministries, such as the Ministry of Finance.

(4) The importance of early attention to designing and installing a reporting system on key variables so as to inform fully and on time the semiannual reviews of progress.

TABLE 2
3249 – Zambia, Basic Ed Sec Inv Prg
Project Status Report Date: **6/30/99**

Region:	AFR	Country:	ZAMBIA			Sector:	EP	Lending Instr:	APL
Prg Obj Cat:	PA	EA Cat:	C	PTI?	N	NGO?	N	Resettlement?	N

LOAN INFORMATION

Agree Type	L/C/G No.	Orig Amt	Rev'd Amt	Currency Indicator	Prod Line	Signing Date	Effective Date	Suppl Prj ID
IDA	31900	28.50 (SDR)			PE	5/11/99		

Total Original Amount (SDR):	28.50	Total Revised Amount (SDR):	0.00

COFINANCING INFORMATION

Agency	Board Amount ($M)	Current Amount ($M)
Total	0.00	0.00

Guarantee Type:	Guarantee Amount ($M):

This form is part of: **Initial Summary**
Read together with:

( ) Aide-memoire	Mission End Date:	This Form PSR Date:	5/20/99
( ) BTO memo of:	Months since last mission:	Last Form PSR Date:	
( ) Follow-up letter of:	Next mission planned:		

SUPERVISION EFFORT	Total Staff-Weeks	Total $000	Field Staff-Weeks	Field $000	As of 6/30/99
Current FY - Planned	4.40	13.25			
Current FY - Actual	7.70	25.67	0.00	0.00	
Board through preceding FY	0.00	0.00	0.00	0.00	
Total Actual	7.70	25.67	0.00	0.00	

UPI No.	Mission Member	Division	No. of Fld Days	Role or Specialization	Previous Mission